Different Diagnoses, Similar Experiences

Different Diagnoses, Similar Experiences: Narratives of Mental Health, Addiction Recovery and Dual Diagnosis

EDITED BY

MICHAEL JOHN NORTON
HSE Office of Mental Health Engagement and Recovery, Ireland

AND

OLIVER JOHN CULLEN
HSE Mental Health Services, Ireland

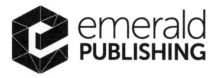

United Kingdom – North America – Japan – India – Malaysia – China

Emerald Publishing Limited
Emerald Publishing, Floor 5, Northspring, 21-23 Wellington Street, Leeds LS1 4DL.

First edition 2024

Reprints and permissions service
Contact: www.copyright.com

British Library Cataloguing in Publication Data
A catalogue record for this book is available from the British Library

ISBN: 978-1-80455-849-2 (Print)
ISBN: 978-1-80455-848-5 (Online)
ISBN: 978-1-80455-850-8 (Epub)

Printed and bound by CPI Group (UK) Ltd, Croydon, CR0 4YY

INVESTOR IN PEOPLE

Contents

Part 2 Mental Health

Part 3 Addiction

Part 4 Dual Diagnosis

List of Figures

Chapter 1

Chapter 2

Chapter 3

Chapter 5

Chapter 25

About the Editors

Michael John Norton is a Recovery and Engagement Programme Lead with the HSE Mental Health Engagement and Recovery Office, based in the Republic of Ireland. He is also a Part-time Lecturer at University College Cork and a Dissertation Supervisor at RCSI Graduate School of Healthcare Management. In his role, Michael John has responsibility for the implementation of recovery-orientated practice across the entire Irish mental health services. One such aspect of this is Michael's involvement in the development of Peer Support Workers in the said service. He is also module co-ordinator for a module exploring mental health policy and practice with University College Cork as part of the QQI level six award in Mental Health in the Community. Additionally, Michael is also a lifelong learner and is currently engaged in a number of programmes of study at postgraduate level. When Michael is not working and studying, he spends his time being an advocate for mental health and evidence-based practice through his involvement in the peer-review process for several high-impact journals and in being a member of several working groups nationally and internationally looking at areas such as co-production, family recovery and trauma. Michael is also an early career researcher whose research interests include peer support work, co-production, patient and public involvement, recovery education, mental health and personal/social recovery.

Oliver John Cullen has lived experience of dual diagnosis – a combination of both mental health and addiction challenges. He is a passionate advocate for recovery in his community where he has worked and volunteered extensively. His roles include Recovery Education Facilitator, Peer Support Worker, Peer Advocacy through engagement with forums and a *Public and Patient Involvement Consultant* on several research projects, covering areas that include peer support, co-production and service change. Oliver has spoken extensively and openly about his lived experience both on radio and a variety of mental health conferences. Oliver's mission is to encourage change within services and wider society by encouraging others to speak about their own challenges and experiences in order to reduce stigma. He has qualifications relating to peer support and addictions from Dublin City University and the Institute of Technology Carlow, now South East Technological University. For Oliver, the purpose of this edited book is to allow others to speak about their own recovery journey in order to demonstrate that recovery is possible for those who choose such a path. He hopes you enjoy, learn and experience hope as you read this book.

About the Contributors

Anonymous 1 (Chapter 12) – A human following a deeply reflective life, breaking patterns, who is a jack of all trades but master of none, deeply interested in humans and helping and learning to rest.

Anonymous 2 (Chapter 21) – Anonymous 2 is a 28-year-old male from the south of Ireland. After secondary school, he studied French, mathematics, and psychology in NUI Maynooth [now Maynooth University] for a year. He dropped out of NUI Maynooth after the year and started working as a security guard for five years and then as a Heavy Goods Vehicle [HGV] driver for a further two and a half years. Now, he is in recovery and is currently upskilling with the hope of soon entering back into full employment.

Arlene is a 38-year-old from Co. Kilkenny. She has pretty much lived there all her life and loved it. She was surrounded by her family in a village that, as a teenager, she couldn't wait to escape from! But priorities shift as you grow older and she couldn't be happier than where she is now, surrounded by all this support from a loving family – in all aspects of her life, not just in recovery. She is still trying to find the new Arlene after the past 15 years or so. She keeps to herself but is very social with people she knows and trusts. She was good fun and friendly, although sometimes her face might tell you differently as she was a very deep thinker, and always had been. She liked to know the answers to everything and never liked to wonder for too long before finding out. Psychology and behaviour fascinated her, and she had studied it, although this wasn't the area she worked in. Like most mothers, she lived and breathed for her kids, mentioning that they kept her going. She expressed being very proud of them and proud of herself for who they were so far. She stated her love for animals, mentioning she had six pets at the moment and counting. She liked to think she was kind-hearted and liked to help people if at all possible.

Kate Byrne is an example of, and advocate of recovery in the community. She is involved in 12-step programmes and supports others in recovery. She recently completed a Diploma in Training and Development in Sustainable Workplaces, including Equality and Addiction Studies. She is currently studying for a Master's in Business Administration. She is a mother to three wonderful children who are flourishing in a loving home. Kate believes that the experiences and struggles we survive in life, add golden threads to the tapestry of our lives. Thus, allowing us to enrich the lives of those around us.

Mark Coyle is a 45-year-old and from Ballymun in North Dublin. He was a Professional Dry Cleaner and enjoyed working in this area for the last 25 years. He has a beautiful daughter who is nine years of age and her name is Eva. Eva is his hope and recovery journey as she shone the light on him especially when the days got hard with her amazing smile and the fun elements she brings to his life and that is how he knows now that hope and recovery are possible. He has been in recovery for the last six years from alcohol and suffered from anxiety due to alcohol intake and other stresses for the last 20 years. He has hope now, and telling his story helps his recovery and hopes it inspires others.

Claire Foy in 2014, at the age of 34, entered the workforce. Having been influenced by the frustration of her own experience and a drive to support others who were struggling with mental health and addiction, Claire has been working in the charity and NGO sector with marginalised groups since that point. She has experience as a frontline worker in low-threshold settings with marginalised populations and later in governance, policy and advocacy roles in several national charities. She is hoping to return to education to complete her post-graduate studies and she has long-term goals that include continuing a career path that enables her to influence social justice and health care reforms for marginalised populations, in particular for those experiencing, homelessness, addiction and those within the prison system.

Andrew C. Grundy is currently working as a Lived Experience Researcher in the School of Health Sciences, University of Manchester, UK. He is also the Lived Experience Research Lead at the Mental Health Policy Research Unit, University College London. Andrew's PhD explored service user perspectives on and experiences of risk and its assessment and management in an acute psychiatric setting. His main research interests are in understanding concepts of 'mental health' and mental health service provision from service user/survivor perspectives. He's also interested in critical approaches to public involvement and co-production in research.

Laura Hardiman is 30 years old and lives in Wexford. She has spent the last 6 years building a recovery lifestyle that keeps her feeling connected to herself, others and her place in the world. She likes a balanced life of being outdoors and sitting on the couch, watching horror films and reading poetry in equal measure. Her current focus is on community and working towards social recovery. She tries to always keep her mind open and changeable, but one thing she knows for sure is the healing power of relationships.

John had been in recovery from addiction and mental health challenges for two decades. His journey hadn't always been easy but deemed it undoubtedly worthwhile and meaningful. Currently, he is working in mental health services, where he utilised his lived experience to inform his practice alongside his professional competencies. He expressed hope that his narrative, along with the many other stories of hope in the book, would be helpful.

Jack Kilkenny is a recovering addict and alcoholic. He reflected on how his life used to revolve around drinking and drugs, focusing primarily on living for the weekends. However, he stated that it wasn't like that anymore. He is a family man who prioritised hard work and lived and breathed recovery. He emphasised the importance of recovery in his life, stating that without it, he would have nothing.

Jenny Langley is a passionate and positive-minded peer support worker, mother of three, and former Marketing professional who spent several months in hospital in 2021, confronting the damage caused by years of grief, trauma and depression. Determined to turn things around she embarked on a journey of personal growth, healing, self-compassion and resilience. Through regular psychology sessions, Compassion-Focused Therapy (CFT), Cognitive-Behavioural Therapy (CBT), Wellness Recovery Action Planning (WRAP) and peer support, she transformed her mental health. Jenny recently obtained her Certificate in Peer Support Working in Mental Health from DCU, solidifying her commitment to helping others self-determine their mental health journeys. Believing in the transformative power of sharing stories, she hopes to empower others to embrace resilience and find hope in their own narratives.

James (Jimmy) Lewis is the Founder of Pleaze. A mobile app that is dedicated to tackling issues with mental health and addiction with innovative approaches. After struggling with mental health and addiction issues for the majority of his life, his mission is to help as many as possible.

Michaela Mc Daid is an Ecotherapy Facilitator, Writer and Speaker from the Northwest of Ireland. Ecotherapy is where her personal and professional life met and everything fell into place. As an avid diarist since childhood, Michaela doesn't know how to be in this world without writing about being in this world and is currently writing her memoir. As for the 'speaking' part, chatting comes very naturally to this middle-aged Irish woman.

L. McGowan is currently employed as a family support practitioner in Ireland. She is a graduate of Atlantic Technological University, Mayo where she completed a degree in Social Care. She also completed a Certificate in Peer Support Practice. Her area of interest is trauma and she is currently studying for a Professional Doctorate in Health, Education, and Society where she intends to explore the topic of gender-based violence. She is a dedicated volunteer with much experience in various charities and organisations. Her credentials, work experience and volunteering show her unwavering dedication to the health and social care areas.

Paul is a 58-year-old father of four and is in recovery from substance abuse. He is at present finishing an Access year at University College Dublin as a mature student and will start a Degree course in Sociology and Social Policy in the autumn. His previous career was in the hospitality sector as Head Chef in many Dublin establishments. He has now returned to studies and has a particular interest in early education and prevention through community endeavours and education for young people regarding addiction issues. He has written of his own battle with addiction here and its subsequent effect on his mental health in a frank and open manner.

Amy Ryan is living in Cork City. She enjoys shopping, drinking coffee and people-watching in 'town'. She is often found chatting on the phone with her friends and sister, travelling to new places and coming up with new ideas.

Shay works as an Engineer and, previous to this, a creative carpenter with a keen eye for detail. Having grown up as a lonely child until his teenage years in Kilkenny, he was involved in numerous sports as an active child. He is passionate about music and running which keeps his body and mind active and healthy and is generally an active person. He is a caring person who is always there to offer support and help others. His goal in life is to be an inspirational father figure, support his family and keep pounding the pavement until his body gives in and then complains about it.

The Eternal Student (Chapter 9) is a person no better or no worse than anyone else.

Acknowledgements

Michael John Norton
This book is the result of Ollie's and my passion for recovery. I am, at the time of writing, nine years in recovery from mental health challenges. I have achieved many things in these nine years. Including this book. However, none of this would have been possible without the support of certain people in my life. Firstly, to my Mum – Mary Ann and my Dad – John, you both have supported me throughout my life in many different ways. You continue to be a source of knowledge, a source of love and support to this day despite the challenges life brings. For all your support over the years and for the years to come, I want to thank you dearly. To my brothers Paddy and Eddie, I know I said this before but my ability to reach the stars academically would not be possible without you both taking the slack off me and working hard on the farm. For taking on that extra burden, thank you. To Louise, my sister-in-law. The final few months of making this book must have been some of the hardest times in our family's life. For supporting Mam and Paddy in particular, thank you. To Sophie and Cody – my godchildren, this book is dedicated to you. I hope you never have to face anything like what the contributors faced in this book, but if you do, I hope this book can provide some comfort. For being the light of my life, the reason I breathe, and the motivator to achieve all I can achieve in life I thank you and I love you both dearly.

To my friends, Linda and Dwayne, once again, I have completed another book and yet again this has resulted in less time being spent with you doing the stuff we love. For understanding why I need to do this, and for making that sacrifice and being there, I thank you. To my co-editor Ollie, thank you for being my friend, for being my sounding board every time something goes wrong and for your enthusiasm across this journey, I thank you and I feel blessed to call you my friend.

Finally, but by no means least, thank you to the contributors of this edited text. Without your generosity in sharing your experiences with us, this book would have never been possible. Your stories are awe-inspiring and hopeful and I hope the reader gets as much inspiration from your narratives as Ollie and I did over the course of the making of this text. Finally, to the audience of this book, I hope this book is not only a source of information but also a source of hope to you and your family and proof that with hard work and dedication, recovery is possible.

Oliver John Cullen

The idea of writing this book came from a conversation between two peers. That is myself and my co-editor Michael. It was born from an idea that recovery is not only evident in our day-to-day interactions, but it is absolutely attainable, even when it seems insurmountable. Myself and Michael have achieved many things against the odds, and we felt like it was time to show others through publication that recovery is difficult, it's harrowing, it can make or break you, it's often born out of trauma, existential crisis and can really bring us to the brink of our semblance of self. However, once the recovery path begins to take on a life of its own, we achieve many, many things, peace, love, harmony, balance, intuition, identity, purpose, honesty, integrity, a life of your own choosing and so much more.

Recovery is an exploratory journey of self-discovery, that has many branching paths, some paths don't have the answer, but that's ok! We learn on this journey that nothing is linear and nothing is wasted. To not try is to miss the opportunity to discover what 'may' or 'may not' work for you. I personally have lifted every rock, looked through every crack and stepped forward when I felt it was right, paused, reflected and looked for guidance and support when I wasn't as sure.

The ironic thing is that during the writing of this book, I wasn't so sure. I struggled and I lost hope. I was admitted to the psychiatric services for 10 weeks, but I needed that additional support. I needed that clinical help. I pushed many people away, and I lost hope, but others did not. They kept in contact; they told me that '*it was ok not to be ok*' even when my ego told me that I don't need anyone to help me. When I finally relinquished the responsibility of recovering on my own, I started to see that I too had lost my identity, I had lost my passion for life through disconnection and emotional turmoil. Then through that re-connection, I became re-enchanted and invigorated with life. Consequently, I have grown and I am humbled by my experiences and the people who continue in silence to grow with me.

To all of those people, I want to say thanks, thank you for telling me, I am enough, I am valued, I am loved. And most of all I couldn't have done this without you.

To Demelza and Olivia, you are the light and hope that I carry inside of me, without you my life would be devoid of all meaning. To my wonderful mother Triona, you showed me how to be kind, to care, allowed me to express my feelings without judgement, and loved me as I believe no other mother could love a son. I love you with all my heart. To my father Ollie Snr, you showed me how to live with dignity and self-respect, and silently supported me all my life. I want you to know I am eternally grateful, and I love you and I hope I make you proud. To my sister Corinna, thank you for looking out for me in my formative years, never questioning my fear of the dark, embracing me and telling me, everything was going to be ok. My love for you is never-ending…

To my co-editor Michael, you hold the same values as I do, you have the same passion and in-depth personal experiences as me, you supported me so much with this book, giving me the time and space, I needed to heal for those months in hospital, and the work we did on the book when you came to visit kept me focused on my recovery, thank you.

To my friends, Karly, Murf and Woodsy, I love you all dearly and thank you for being like brothers to me. To my friend Agatha, who gave me the opportunity to be heard, to be seen and her vigilance for my wellbeing has kept me safe many, many times.

To my team in St Pats, you gave me encouragement, support, empathy and clinic expertise and are an integral part of my recovery. Thank you.

To my additional friends whom I don't have the word count to thank personally! I want you to know that you gave me respect and that's all I needed, and I value you as I value my closest allies.

To the friends/family who have left this mortal coil. I think about you every day, and you are forever in my heart.

And would also like to thank the contributors to the book, your courage and strength have resonated with me on such a deep level, that can't be explained in any textbook. I truly am humbled that you have put your voice forward to support the premise of this book and to inspire others that are on or contemplating their own journey of recovery.

Part 1

Context

Chapter 1

Contextual and Personal Introduction to the Text

Michael John Norton[a] and Oliver John Cullen[b]

[a] *HSE Office of Mental Health Engagement and Recovery, Ireland*
[b] *HSE Mental Health Services, Ireland*

Abstract

This, the first chapter of this text provides an introduction to a social world that is constructed through cultural attitudes, with a long history of the so-called '*insane*' or deviants being excluded from society. In many cases, this was due to their behaviour resulting from an addiction issue, mental ill health or as is often the case, both. The chapter begins with an introduction to what led to the conceptualisation of this text. Once this occurs, the interplay between the '*normal*' and the deviant, as discussed above, is played through an examination of the cultural perceptions of both mental health and addiction. In addition, to support this, a brief historical timeline of mental health, addiction and dual diagnosis is described and visually depicted. Finally, the chapter concludes with an introduction to both editors of this text who then describe what will be discussed in the chapters that follow.

Keywords: Addiction; dual diagnosis; history; mental health; recovery; stigma

1.1. Introduction

Compared to that of addiction services, the application of personal recovery and associated models in mental health discourse has only occurred relatively recently (International Mental Health Collaborating Network, n.d.). Recovery was not

Different Diagnoses, Similar Experiences:
Narratives of Mental Health, Addiction Recovery and Dual Diagnosis, 3–18
Copyright © 2024 by Michael John Norton and Oliver John Cullen
Published under exclusive licence by Emerald Publishing Limited
doi:10.1108/978-1-80455-848-520241001

heard of in mental health service provision until the seminal work of William Anthony, who defined the concept in 1993. Here, Anthony defines recovery as:

> [...] a deeply personal, unique process of changing one's attitudes, values, feelings, goals, skills and/or roles. It is a way of living a satisfying, hopeful and contributing life even with the limitations caused by illness. Recovery involves the development of new meaning and purpose in one's life as one grows beyond the catastrophic effects of mental illness.

Since 1993, we have learned a lot in terms of both mental health and addiction recovery and the similarities between them. For instance, both of them rely on the power of peer support to enable and maintain the life transformation required to recover. Both view recovery, not as an end destination, but as a lifelong journey with many peaks and troughs rely on the personal responsibility of each individual to abstain and continuously work at their own recovery throughout the lifecycle of an individual.

This text was born out of a common interest for both editors of this book, the first editor [MJN] has lived experience of mental health difficulties and familial experience of addiction challenges. The other editor [OJC] has lived experience of both mental health and addiction challenges. Chapter 1 of this text aims to provide some contextual information relating to the cultural and historical underpinnings of mental health, addiction and dual diagnosis challenges within our society. The chapter is divided into a number of sections, each exploring parts of this chapter's aim. Section 1.2 explores the cultural perceptions of mental health and addiction. This is vital in understanding how society views mental health and addiction issues as it will provide further clarity into the lack of understanding of these complex issues. Section 1.3 provides a brief history of mental health, addiction and dual diagnosis. This will be carried out by analysing them separately first before combining the key points in Fig. 1.1. Section 1.4 introduces the editors to the audience, followed by Section 1.5 which details the structure of the book. Finally, Section 1.6 concludes the chapter by providing a brief synopsis of what was discussed before focussing attention on Chapter 2. Section 1.2 will now be presented.

1.2. Cultural Perceptions of Mental Health and Addiction

The concept of culture is abstract and refers to a set of beliefs, norms and values of a particular group of people that form part of society (Department of Health & Human Services, 2001). It is important to examine culture as it relates to health care as it is intrinsically linked with service quality (Mannion & Davies, 2018). For example, increased awareness of the importance of culture within the healthcare setting has led to the facilitation of better communication pathways between service providers and those utilising the services (Kaihlanen et al., 2019). Here, a discussion regarding the impact of culture on both mental health and addiction will be presented. It is important to understand the nuances within the perception

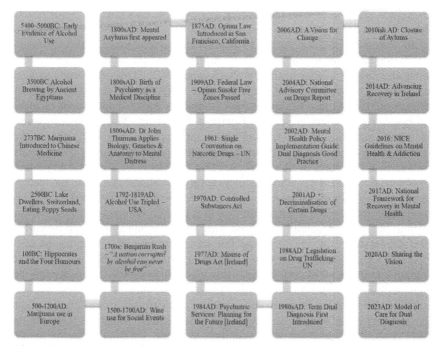

Fig. 1.1.   Mental Health, Addiction and Dual Diagnosis Throughout the Ages – A Detailed Timeline.

of both types of challenges within society at present so that an acute awareness of the sensitivities and stereotypical nature of each type of challenge can make a difference in recovery outcomes for such individuals.

1.2.1. Cultural Perceptions of Mental Health

The concept of culture and its association with the diagnosis, treatment and overall recovery journey of those with a mental health challenge is quite strong (Al-Krenawi, 2019). Culture has impacted mental health discourse for thousands of years. For example, before the mid-1800s, mental ill health or deviant behaviours or phenomena were thought to have been rooted in the area of religion and spirituality and as a result treated in such a manner that represents this flow of thinking (Norton, 2022). In some developing world cultures, this conclusion is still logical as the cause of mental ill health (Ahmad & Koncsol, 2022). This disparity of sources of mental distress and its true inner meaning has caused differences in the way those appearing to be in mental distress are treated. For those regions that still actively believe in a spiritual or religious cause for mental distress, the nature of the religious belief used to support and cope with the distress influences the long-term recovery outcomes of the individual affected (Lucchetti et al., 2021). In addition, in an article focussed on the cultural differences in perspectives of voice-hearing, Parker (2014) found that the culture influenced how these individuals lived with their voices. For example, as a sense of a nonviolent mind, a source of closeness to God and so on.

In westernised societies, although mental health and physical health are intrinsically linked, there remains a lack of information and indeed understanding when it comes to mental health (Mohankumar, 2022). This often leads to dual comorbidity as the individual not only has to suffer the life-changing effects of their condition but also the stereotypes, prejudices and misconceptions of mental health from others in society (Corrigan & Watson, 2002). This can result in stigma occurring within mental health service provision. The term stigma describes the behaviour of devaluing, discrediting and/or shaming based solely on personal attributes or characteristics that the victim of stigma may possess (Subu et al., 2021). In a study examining rates of stigma overtime for mental health challenges such as depression, and schizophrenia, Pescosolido et al. (2021) found that although there was a decrease in stigma for depression over a 20-year period, the sense of volatility in those with schizophrenia and related psychotic illnesses increased by 15.7% during this same time period. These results suggest that although mental distress is becoming more acceptable as part of the human condition within our society, this assumption is not the reality for the more enduring and serious mental health challenges such as schizophrenia and other psychotic-based illnesses. As a result of such stigma, many consequences can arise for those who use services at the centre of such dilemmas (Geraldo da Silva et al., 2020). Such consequences include shame, self-blame, discrimination and isolation (Latoo et al., 2021).

Consequently, with the rise of the recovery movement, came the realisation that those with mental health challenges have a unique knowledge set which could only be gained from living through an experience of mental ill health (Norton, 2022). The realisation of this lived experience – known technically as experiential knowledge – brought with it a number of initiatives which have been known to reduce stigma towards those who have had a mental health challenge. Such initiatives include peer support work, co-production, recovery education and peer academics to name just a few. Unfortunately, despite this realisation, a recent study reported in *The Guardian* by De Jong (2023) suggests that stigma has increased for those with a psychotic disorder since the year 1990. As such, the report leads one to suggest that although positive change has occurred in recent years relating to culture, stigma and mental health, more work is needed in order to resolve the inequities experienced by people who use services as a result of their mental health challenge. In addition, this has raised further calls for an examination of culturally associated health beliefs and how they impact the treatment received by individuals within the mental health system (Jimenez et al., 2012).

1.2.2. Cultural Perceptions of Addiction

The perspectives surrounding addiction challenges differ significantly depending on the person asked and the culture in which they were born and reared. For instance, in Irish culture, it is quite normal within this society to have a drink after the end of a hard day's work, at weekends and for major events within the lifecycle such as births, baptism, holy communion and so on. However, despite this cultural norm, alcohol abuse is linked to a number of diseases and is associated with approximately three million deaths per annum globally (World Health Organization, 2022). Alcohol and associated pathologies also have an economic, familial, organisational and self-destructive impact, which has led to calls to review the legality and social acceptability of the substance across the world (Jankhotkaew et al., 2022).

Of equal concern is the upward trend of the use of powerful stimulants, such as MDMA and crack cocaine ['free base'] in our society. For instance, Ireland currently ranks 80 per capita for alcohol consumption, with a dependency rate of 3.8% (Wisevoter, 2023). Economically, the resulting service needs to be created due to this is approximately €2.3 billion to the Irish economy (O'Halloran, 2018). Alarmingly, the Department of Health (2019) noted that 26.4% of those aged 15 years and over have used an illegal, illicit substance at some point during their lifetime. This knowledge may suggest that a good percentage of these individuals have made a conscientious decision to consume such substances, despite the prior knowledge relating to the legality of its use and the potential harms that can occur as a result of the misuse of the substance. The usage of certain substances has increased at an alarming rate (Mongan et al., 2021). For example, cocaine use has increased by 7% in males aged 25–34 years within an 18-year period leading to 2020.

As already identified for mental health, stigma also has an extremely negative impact on those in recovery from substance misuse challenges, particularly towards issues of trust and fear. In addition, to societal stigma, negative attitudes towards those with substance misuse issues can even occur amongst the individuals taking the substance. For instance, individuals whose substance of abuse is alcohol may not consider themselves an addict and instead refer to those with other types of addiction negatively as their addiction is more normally accepted than, for example, an opiate addiction. Such stigmatising assumptions can affect the recovery journey of those in addiction, particularly if there is a need to take supplemental medication to maintain stability and recovery. Stigma can come in many forms including from society to professionals to self-stigma (Subu et al., 2021). Stigma, particularly from professionals, can affect the quality of care received (Degnan et al., 2021). Language is also an important factor in the treatment of those with addiction challenges. For example, the use of derogatory terms such as 'addict' and 'abuser' can infer negative connotations onto the individual by self and community leading to stigmatisation (Quigley, 2022; Shi et al., 2022).

However, unlike the perpetual effects, addiction has on an individual and their surrounding social world, addiction as a pathophysiology, a trauma, does not discriminate between social or ethnic classes. There are many conceptual models that support our understanding of recovery from addiction. For example, Canadian Physician, Dr Gabor Mate claims that the source of addiction is not to be found in one's genes, but in early childhood experiences (Mate, 2018). Whatever reason an individual chooses to use an addictive substance, that experience, for certain individuals increases the release of dopamine, providing a rewarding sensation which leads to repetition of use in order to replicate the euphoric feelings achieved as a result. A *New York Times* article describes the devastating impact of the opioid crisis in America. One individual vividly describes '*remember[ing the] feeling like [they were] exhaling from holding [their] breath for [their] whole life*'. Another individual suggested that the euphoric feelings achieved from substance misuse were '*like being hugged by Jesus*' (Sinha, 2018). Previous understandings of addiction would point towards detox, with perhaps a medical intervention and recovery support groups as a continued source of peer support and a reminder of the challenges that were once prevalent in the individual's life. But now we know there are many alternate routes that can be taken, including education, therapeutic interventions, and pharmacological support (e.g. methadone or buprenorphine for opiate maintenance). The individual also has choice and autonomy around their recovery pathways.

In terms of support around recovery for addiction, there are also multiple avenues a person in addiction can follow towards recovery based on what they feel works best for them. For example, SMART Recovery centres on the principles of choice and autonomy, delivered through a four-point programme:

1.   Building and maintaining motivation,
2.   Coping with urges,
3.   Managing thoughts, feelings, and behaviours,
4.   Living a balanced life.

(SMART Recovery, 2022)

SMART stands for Self-Management and Recovery Training. It is an approach based on cognitive behavioural therapy which aims to assist individuals to achieve and maintain recovery. This is achieved through the programme empowering individuals to use the tools and practices promoted by SMART in their own lives, including the use of self-empowering and destigmatising language.

Another model: Alcoholics Anonymous [AA] promotes a different perspective on recovery through a 12-step programme which suggests that the individual is ultimately powerless over their addiction and relies on a higher power to achieve and maintain recovery. The model is traditionally based on the Christian faith and belief in God. Over time this has changed to be inclusive of many faiths and spiritual beliefs. Unlike SMART, AA often utilises terms such as alcoholic or addict to describe the individuals who use this service for recovery as it sees addiction as a disease, that can be cured using the programme. According to Drugs. ie (2018), stigma also comes into play within the way society views addiction to illicit substances – a crime. There is evidence to suggest that addiction should be viewed as a healthcare issue and as such, how it is viewed should be pathological in nature as a result. According to The Gateway Foundation (2023), using the judicial system to solve the addiction challenge does not work as it is a disease of the brain that has societal consequences, and not vice versa. The approach used currently [the judicial system] reinforces stigma and keeps individuals in a vicious cycle of trauma with little hope of obtaining and maintaining recovery. This is evident through the Dillon et al. (2022) report which identified that in 2022, 70%

of inmates in prison services have an underlying substance misuse challenge. Viewing addiction as a healthcare issue does offer possible solutions, including detox programmes, therapeutic intervention and group support which are currently undervalued in the judicial system.

1.3. A Brief History of Mental Health, Addiction and Dual Diagnosis

Mental health and addiction have had a long, but turbulent history due to their ever-changing nature relating to understanding the root cause of each issue (O'Mahony, 2020; Tasca et al., 2012). This section introduces a brief historical context of three separate, but interconnecting concepts: mental health, addiction and dual diagnosis. This is carried out in order to provide some context of the journey taken by services towards recovery: the philosophical concept and movement. A visual summary of the interplay between the history behind each of these three concepts is depicted in Fig. 1.1, with further description provided from Sections 1.3.1 to 1.3.3 inclusive below.

1.3.1. Mental Health

Since the dawn of time, scholars have searched for the meaning behind mental health problems. This search into the abyss was ultimately to find a suitable cure that would rid the person of the origins of their distress. Over time, different perspectives on the cause of mental health challenges accumulated in scholarship relating to this area. In the century or so before the life of Christ, a Greek physician by the name of Hippocrates attributed madness to an imbalance of one or more of the four humours of the body: blood, yellow bile, black bile and phlegm (Ross & Margolis, 2018). However, this idea of four humours and the creation of illness through an imbalance within the human body would eventually subside as more spiritual and moral explanations for mental distress began to emerge. The idea of mental distress occurring as a result of demonic possession, led many under the catholic faith to undergo exorcisms and other malpractices in a desperate bid to expel the demonic force or spirit from the physical body and return it to a place of homeostasis. However, by the mid-1800s, knowledge pertaining to mental distress began to revert to the same logic as Hippocrates imbalance of humour which occurred a millennium earlier.

In the 18th century, the biomedical model began as Dr John Thurman proceeded to apply the sciences of biology, genetics and anatomy to the phenomenon of mental distress (Dickinson, 1990). Instead of the four humours, such imbalance was electrical or chemical in nature, often with residual effects of the ventricles or brain structure itself. This led to the birth of psychiatry as a medical discipline and the relocation of those deemed mad into asylums. These asylums would later be known for their deplorable living conditions and inhumane acts of treatment to correct the imbalance or deal with the changing pathology as it alters brain structure. In the 1900s, medical advances in the field of psychiatry and neuroscience led to the cessation of barbaric treatments associated with being mentally unwell in favour of psychotropic medications (Norton, 2022). However, electroconvulsive therapy remained and is still viewed as a viable treatment option today. What also remained were the asylums, where cohorts of mentally unwell individuals would live out their days under the confines of the walls of these buildings. Within an Irish service context, a policy document was released in 1984 by the Department of Health which aimed to end the existence of the traditional asylums (Norton, 2019). *'The Psychiatric Services – Planning for the Future'* (Department of Health, 1984) would ultimately fail to reach the traction required for organisational change resulting in the continuation of this way of working until after the publication of *'A Vision for Change'* in 2006 (Department of Health, 2006).

Although not enacted fully until much later, *'A Vision for Change'* has helped create the philosophical, structural and organisational change required to support recovery. The recovery promoted in this document and context does not relate to the alleviation of symptoms of distress, rather it is about building a good life even with the presence of mental ill health. Additionally, the policy caused the traditional asylums of the time to close down, the creation of multi-disciplinary teams and the use of recovery as an empirical concept and as a movement, which resulted in the employment of those with lived experience to co-produce service design, delivery and evaluation. In 2014, Ireland signed up for Implementing Recovery through Organisational Change [ImROC]. A campaign that was supported by the University of Nottingham aimed at deconstructing the organisational barrier to recovery. This partnership continued until 2017 when Irish mental health services launched their own framework for recovery: *'A National Framework for Recovery in Mental Health'*. Here, recovery was said to be embedded if four principles were realised by the service – (1) the centrality of the service user's lived experience, (2) the co-production of recovery-orientated services, (3) an organisational commitment to recovery and (4) recovery-orientated learning and practice (Health Service Executive, 2017).

At the time of writing, the recovery movement has grown phenomenally. In Irish services, there are recovery-orientated practitioners representing all parts of the system – from peer management through Area Leads, Recovery Co-Ordinators, members of the Mental Health Engagement and Recovery Office, to peer education staff/teams and Family/Peer Support Workers. Internationally, Eastern European countries are beginning to move away from the biomedical mechanisms of service delivery and are expanding their knowledge base to include recovery. In essence, the history of mental health can be viewed in three main eras, Hippocrates four humours and the revitalisation of same through the biomedical model in later years, the time of spiritual awakeness and control and the move towards recovery and lived experience as a knowledge set.

1.3.2. Addiction

Like that of mental health, the history of addiction is a fascinating one. The phenomenon is said to be thousands of years old. The history of addiction is so vast that to explain it in detail goes beyond the focus of this text. However, a focus here will be on the historical context of three addictive substances: opium, alcohol and cocaine, in the hopes of providing insight into how addiction as a neurological and social process is thousands of years old. For instance, fossil evidence dating back to the Neolithic Period [12,000 – 2,000 BC], confirms the presence and use of such substances in prehistoric society (Evolve, n.d.). However, whether they were used for recreational or medicinal purposes remains a mystery.

For example, the poppy plant has been used to produce the substance: opium, a potent substance often used in medicine as an opiate to treat severe pain. However, it is also known for its addictive properties, particularly through its use in recreational and highly regulated medicinal products such as heroin, oxycontin and codeine. As its addictive properties became realised by wider society, demand for the substance increased, particularly in Europe and China (Dea Museum, n.d.).

Opium is not the only substance that has both a practical and harm-inducing use in our society. Take, for instance, cocaine. Cocaine was first introduced as an ingredient in the beverage 'Coca-Cola'. Additionally, it also had medicinal value, being used for the treatment of several disorders including depression, and asthma (Holstege et al., 2021). However, due to its highly addictive and somewhat fatal properties, eventually, cocaine was legislated alongside that of opium in the Dangerous Drugs Act UK (1920) (Legislation.Gov.UK, 1920). Another example is that of alcohol. Alcohol was created in ancient Mesopotamia to solve poor water quality attained from the environment (Namou, n.d.). Consequently, alcohol also proved to be addictive and as such in later years was also legislated against. Despite this, to this day, alcohol is still a legal substance that can be used to excess by some individuals in society. As noted above, a complete history of addiction goes beyond the scope of this text. However, here, for the purposes of context, examples from across history, as it pertains to opium, cocaine and alcohol will be documented.

From this historical analysis, it is evident that as knowledge increased about the potent effects of these substances, so did their integration into the social world. Take, for instance, alcohol. Evidence suggests that the use of alcoholic substances, like wine, dates back to the period 5,400–5,000 B.C. This has been verified through the process of carbon dating (Harutyunyan & Malfeito-Ferreira, 2022). In 3,500 BC, the use of alcohol remained with evidence suggesting that alcohol was being brewed by the ancient Egyptians (Maksoud et al., 1994). In 2,500 BC, evidence suggests that a lake dweller in Switzerland ate poppy seeds for the effects of opium (Montagu, 1966). Later in 2,737 BC, Marijana was first referenced as being used within ancient Chinese medicine. However, the substance failed to reach Europe till 500 AD (Brande, 2023). It took another 700 years before cannabis was officially documented as being present on this same continent (TD Consultancy, n.d.). Albala (2014) notes the continuous presence of alcohol, particularly wine in Europe between 1,500 and 1,700 AD. In particular, the use of wine at social events like meals. However, with this comes a dichotomy between classes around its use. Other substances, like opium, were also used medicinally during this time for a multitude of conditions ranging from mild to severe (Crumpe, 1793).

In the late 1700s, Benjamin Rush, a founding father of the United States of America was noted challenging the usage of alcohol stating: '*A nation corrupted by alcohol can never be free'.* He maintained and defended this statement till his death. All the while, his defiance was to be of no avail as the amount of alcohol consumed per capita between 1792 and 1819 tripled. Rush was one of the first to identify alcohol addiction as a chronic disease, a notion which eventually became the foundation of many principles of the alcoholic anonymous model of recovery that exists today (Blakley, 2022).

Throughout the 18th century, the presence of addictive substances within society became the norm, with evidence of free trade for medicinal use as legislation regulating such substances remained unavailable at this time. As time went by, and the freelance use of addictive substances became widespread, so too came legislation to regulate the availability and usage of such substances (Crocq, 2007). For example, in 1875, San Francisco introduced a law prohibiting opium dens. Later in 1909, the first federal drug law was enacted introducing opium smoke-free zones (Brecher, 1972). Several decades after this, the then President Nixon brought into law The Controlled Substance Act which for the first-time classified drugs into schedules ranking their potential for abuse (Tarricone, 2020). In 1977, Ireland introduced the Misuse of Drugs Act, which superseded previous acts in response to the growing rates of drug use at that time (Irish Statute Books, 1977). Meanwhile, a global response to the war on drugs began with the United Nations Office of Drugs and Crime introducing changes in law. For instance, in 1961, the Single Convention on Narcotic Drugs noted all controlled substances and merged them into a single drug control agreement (United Nations, 1961). Whereas in 1988, further legislation was passed in response to increased drug trafficking (United Nations, 1988).

Ironically, despite previous efforts to clamp down on drugs through enacting various pieces of legislation, society is starting to notice that drug abuse is more of a societal rather than a legislative issue. For instance, since 2001, Portugal and some American states [Colorado, Washington, California] have decriminalised some illicit substances for use (Ministry of Health [Portugal], 2000; We Change Laws, n.d.). However, the results pertaining to these modern approaches to illicit substances have been described as mixed at best with many other factors noted to be at play, including economics, environment and trauma (Alcohol & Drug Foundation, 2022). As such, at the time of writing, there is still no silver bullet response to this ever-changing landscape.

1.3.3. Dual Diagnosis

The term dual diagnosis, in this context, is a relatively new label, first identified in the 1980s (Hryb et al., 2007), to describe the co-occurrence of mental health and addiction challenges (Fantuzzi & Mezzina, 2020). In the United Kingdom, the recognition of co-occurring disorders within policy began in 2002 with the publication of the '*Mental Health Policy Implementation Guide: Dual Diagnosis Good Practice*' (Health Service Executive, 2023b). Here, for the first time, policy recognised that a mental health disorder and an addiction challenge can occur at the same time and can worsen each respective disorder (Department of Health, 2002).

In Irish services, the first mention of dual diagnosis in policy came with the publication of '*A Vision for Change*' by the Department of Health in 2006 resulting from a report that was commissioned by the National Advisory Committee on Drugs in 2004 (Kelly & Holahan, 2022). At this time, policy took the position that although mental health and addiction challenges can occur in tandem, both types of challenges should be treated as separate entities, leading to services only treating half the original problem (Christie, 2017; Department of Health, 2006). In Australia, in 2015, such siloing of resources towards treatment for mental health and addiction was still in place (New South Wales Ministry of Health, 2015).

In 2016, the National Institute for Health and Clinical Excellence [NICE] concluded that there should not be a separate service for those with dual diagnosis, instead existing services should merge and work together to support the recovery journeys of individuals with co-occurring disorders (Health Service Executive, 2023b). Four years later, in 2020, Ireland updated mental health policy: '*Sharing the Vision*' was published by the Irish Department of Health. This policy retracted the assumption that mental health and addiction should be treated as two separate entities by calling for greater collaboration between both services so that treatment regimens address whole person recovery (Department of Health, 2020; Kelly & Holahan, 2022). In 2023, Ireland, through the work of the HSE National Clinical Programme for Dual Diagnosis, launched the first model of care to address the growing need for services to treat in unison, mental health and addiction challenges (Health Service Executive, 2023a). At the time of writing, this model of care is just being implemented, with much work needed in order to create a service that addresses both the emotional and addictive needs of its citizens. At present, within an Irish context, there are only three services that provide holistic care in this regard: St Patricks Hospital,[1] St. John of Gods hospital[2] and Smarmore Castle.[3]

1.4. Structure of This Book

This text is divided into six interconnecting parts with the aim of showcasing to the reader the similarities and differences in the recovery journey of a person with mental health, substance misuse and dual diagnosis challenges. Additionally, from this, recommendations will be made at the macro, meso and micro levels to support all stakeholders in embracing recovery, regardless of the challenges faced. Part 1 places the book in context with existing literature and policy pertaining to mental health, addiction and dual diagnosis challenges and recovery. Part 2 provides six different recovery narratives relating to mental health challenges. Part 3 provides six new narratives relating to addiction challenges, with Part 4 documenting six more narratives that are associated with living with dual diagnosis.

---

[1]https://www.stpatricks.ie/
[2]https://www.stjohnofgodhospital.ie
[3]https://www.smarmore-rehab-clinic.com

Part 5 uses a thematic analysis style to illustrate and document the similarities and differences between the narratives provided. Following this, it also provides recommendations to both policy and practice for multiple stakeholders, including service providers and service users of the said services. Finally, Part 6 concludes the text by providing a list of helpful resources that health professionals, service users, family members/carers/supporters can use to gather further information and support as needed.

1.5. Concluding Remarks

This chapter aimed to begin providing context and insight into the world of mental health, addiction and dual diagnosis. This was carried out by first examining the cultural perspectives around mental health and addiction. Next, a historical context was provided to document how our awareness and treatment options for such issues changed throughout the course of history. The editors of this text were then introduced through an analysis of their academic and lived experience backgrounds. Finally, the structure of this text was then explained. Chapter 2 will continue providing a contextual background to the text by exploring policy relating to mental health, addiction and dual diagnosis from an Irish and international perspective.

References

Ahmad, S. S., & Koncsol, S. W. (2022). Cultural factors influencing mental health stigma: Perceptions of mental illness (POMI) in Pakistani emerging adults. *Religions, 13*(5), 401. https://doi.org/10.3390/rel13050401

Albala, K. (2014). *Stimulants and intoxicants in Europe, 1500–1700*. Routledge.

Alcohol and Drug Foundation. (2022, November 24). *Overview: Decriminalisation vs legislation*. https://adf.org.au/talking-about-drugs/law/decriminalisation/overview-decriminalisation-legalisation/#:~:text=Decriminalisation%20may%20also%20reduce%20strain,matters%3B%20and%20costs%20of%20imprisonment

Al-Krenawi, A. (2019). The impact of cultural beliefs on mental health diagnosis and treatment. In M. Zangeneh & A. Al-Krenawi (Eds.), *Culture, diversity and mental health – Enhancing clinical practice* (pp. 149–165). Springer Nature.

Anthony, W. A. (1993). Recovery from mental illness: The guiding vision of the mental health service system in the 1990s. *Psychiatric Rehabilitation Journal, 16*, 11–23.

Blakley, L. (2022, July 3). *Historical figures in addiction treatment: Benjamin Rush*. https://www.avenuesrecovery.com/historical-figures-in-addiction-treatment-benjamin-rush/

Brande, L. (2023, February 15). *Marijuana facts, history, and statistics*. https://drugabuse.com/drugs/marijuana/history-statistics/

Brecher, E. M. (1972). *The consumers union report on licit and illicit drugs*. https://www.druglibrary.org/schaffer/library/studies/cu/cu6.htm

Christie, E. (2017). *Better care for people with co-occurring mental health and alcohol/drug use conditions: A guide for commissioners and service providers*. https://assets.publishing.service.gov.uk/government/uploads/system/uploads/attachment_data/file/625809/Co-occurring_mental_health_and_alcohol_drug_use_conditions.pdf

Corrigan, P. W., & Watson, A. C. (2002). Understanding the impact of stigma on people with mental illness. *World Psychiatry, 1*(1), 16–20.

Crocq, M.-A. (2007). Historical and cultural aspects of man's relationship with addictive drugs. *Dialogues in Clinical Neuroscience, 9*(4), 355–361. https://doi.org/10.31887/DCNS.2007.9.4/macrocq

Crumpe, S. (1793). *An inquiry into the nature and properties of opium: Wherein its component principles, mode of operation and use or abuse in particular diseases, are experimentally investigated; and the opinions of former authors on these points impartially examined.* G.G & J. Robinson.

De Jong, E. (2023, July 18). Nobody I've been locked up with in a psychiatric hospital felt proud' of their illness. *The Guardian.* https://www.theguardian.com/commentisfree/2023/jun/19/nobody-ive-ever-been-locked-up-with-in-a-psychiatric-hospital-felt-proud-of-their-illnesses

Dea Museum. (n.d.). *Opium poppy.* https://museum.dea.gov/exhibits/online-exhibits/cannabis-coca-and-poppy-natures-addictive-plants/opium-poppy#:~:text=The%20earliest%20reference%20to%20opium,it%20on%20to%20the%20Egyptians

Degnan, A., Berry, K., Humphrey, C., & Bucci, S. (2021). The relationship between stigma and subjective quality of life in psychosis: A systematic review and meta-analysis. *Clinical Psychology Review, 85,* 102003. https://doi.org/10.1016/j.cpr.2021.102003

Department of Health. (1984). *The psychiatric services – Planning for the future: Report of a study group on the development of the psychiatric services.* https://www.lenus.ie/handle/10147/45556

Department of Health. (2002). *Mental health policy implementation guide: Dual diagnosis good practice guide.* https://webarchive.nationalarchives.gov.uk/ukgwa/20130107105354/http://www.dh.gov.uk/prod_consum_dh/groups/dh_digitalassets/@dh/@en/documents/digitalasset/dh_4060435.pdf

Department of Health. (2006). *A vision for change: Report of the expert group on mental health policy.* https://www.hse.ie/eng/services/publications/mentalhealth/mental-health--a-vision-for-change.pdf

Department of Health. (2019, May 31). *Drugs survey reveals that levels of recent drug use have risen slightly.* https://www.gov.ie/en/press-release/69ecc3-drugs-survey-reveals-that-levels-of-recent-drug-use-have-risenslight/#:~:text=26.4%25%20of%20Irish%20adults%20aged,this%20within%20the%20past%20month

Department of Health. (2020). *Sharing the vision: A mental health policy for everyone.* https://www.gov.ie/pdf/?file=https://assets.gov.ie/76770/b142b216-f2ca-48e6-a551-9c208f1a247.pdf#page=null

Department of Health and Human Services. (2001). *Mental health: Culture, race and ethnicity – A supplement to mental health: A report of the surgeon general.* https://www.ncbi.nlm.nih.gov/books/NBK44243/pdf/Bookshelf_NBK44243.pdf

Dickinson, E. (1990). From madness to mental health: A brief history of psychiatric treatment in the UK from 1800 to the present. *British Journal of Occupational Therapy, 53*(10), 419–424. https://psycnet.apa.org/record/1991-15974-001

Dillon, L., Galvin, B., Guiney, C., Lyons, S., & Millar, S. (2022). *Focal Point Ireland: National Report for 2022 – Prison.* https://www.drugsandalcohol.ie/25265/1/Prisons%20workbook_2022.pdf

Drugs.ie. (2018, February 02). *How stigma can prevent drug users getting the help they need.* https://www.drugs.ie/news/article/you_junkie_you_addict_how_stigma_can_prevent_drug_users_getting_the_help_th

Evolve. (n.d.). *A history of drug use part 1: Prehistory to the classical era.* https://evolvetreatment.com/blog/history-drug-use/

Fantuzzi, C., & Mezzina, R. (2020). Dual diagnosis: A systematic review of the organization of community health services. *International Journal of Social Psychiatry, 66*(3), 300–310. https://doi.org/10.1177/0020764019899975

Geraldo da Silva, A., Baldacara, L., Cavalcante, D. A., Fasanella, N. A., & Palha, A. P. (2020). The impact of mental illness stigma on psychiatric emergencies. *Frontiers in Psychiatry*, *11*, 573. https://doi.org/10.3389/fpsyt.2020.00573

Harutyunyan, M., & Malfeito-Ferreira, M. (2022). The rise of wine among ancient civilisations across the Mediterranean basin. *Heritage*, *5*(2), 788–812. https://doi.org/10.3390/heritage5020043

Health Service Executive. (2017). *A national framework for recovery in mental health 2018–2020.* https://www.getirelandwalking.ie/_files/recovery-framework.pdf

Health Service Executive. (2023a, May 24). *HSE launches new model of care for dual* diagnosis. https://www.hse.ie/eng/services/news/media/pressrel/hse-launches-new-model-of-care-for-dual-diagnosis.html

Health Service Executive. (2023b). *Model of care for people with mental disorders and co-existing substance use disorders (Dual diagnosis).* https://www.hse.ie/eng/about/who/cspd/ncps/mental-health/dual-diagnosis-ncp/dual-diagnosis-model-of-care.pdf

Holstege, C. P., Zhong, Q. X., & Ait-Daoud Tiouririne, N. (2021, November 18). *Cocaine related psychiatric disorders.* https://emedicine.medscape.com/article/290195-overview

Hryb, K., Kirkhart, R., & Talbert, R. (2007). A call for standardized definition of dual diagnosis. *Psychiatry*, *4*(9), 15–16.

International Mental Health Collaborating Network. (n.d.). *History of recovery movement.* https://imhcn.org/bibliography/history-of-mental-health/history-of-recovery-movement/

Irish Statute Books. (1977). *Misuse of drugs act, 1977.* https://www.irishstatutebook.ie/eli/1977/act/12/enacted/en/print.html

Jankhotkaew, J., Casswell, S., Huckle, T., Chaiyasong, S., & Phonsuk, P. (2022). Barriers and facilitators to the implementation of effective alcohol control policies: A scoping review. *International Journal of Environmental Research and Public Health*, *19*(11), 6742. https://doi.org/10.3390/ijerph19116742

Jimenez, D. E., Bartels, S. J., Cardenas, V., Daliwal, S. S., & Alegria, M. (2012). Cultural beliefs and mental health treatment preferences of ethnically diverse older adult consumers in primary care. *American Journal of Geriatric Psychiatry*, *20*(6), 533–542. https://doi.org/10.1097%2FJGP.0b013e318227f876

Kaihlanen, A.-M., Hietapakka, L., & Heponiemi, T. (2019). Increasing cultural awareness: Qualitative study of nurses' perceptions about cultural competence training. *BMC Nursing*, *18*, 38. https://doi.org/10.1186/s12912-019-0363-x

Kelly, K., & Holahan, R. (2022). *Dual recovery: A qualitative exploration of the views of stakeholders working in mental health, substance misuse and homelessness in Ireland on the barriers to recovery for individuals with a dual diagnosis.* https://www.drugsandalcohol.ie/36269/1/Dual-Recovery-Full-Report.pdf

Latoo, J., Mistry, M., Alabdulla, M., Wadoo, O., Jan, F., Munshi, T., Iqbal, Y., & Haddad, P. (2021). Mental health stigma: The role of dualism, uncertainty, causation and treatability. *General Psychiatry*, *34*, e100498. https://doi.org/10.1136/gpsych-2021-100498

Legislation.Gov.UK. (1920). *Dangerous drugs.* https://www.legislation.gov.uk/nisro/1937/97/pdfs/nisro_19370097_en.pdf

Lucchetti, G., Koenig, H. G., & Lucchetti, A. L. G. (2021). Spirituality, religiousness, and mental health: A review of the current scientific evidence. *World Journal of Clinical Cases*, *9*(26), 7620–7631. https://doi.org/10.12998%2Fwjcc.v9.i26.7620

Maksoud, S. A., Hadidi, N. E., & Amer, W. M. (1994). Beer from the early dynasties (3500–3400 cal B.C) of upper Egypt detected by Arche chemical methods. *Vegetation History and Archaeobotany*, *3*(4), 219–224.

Mannion, R., & Davies, H. (2018). Understanding organisational culture for healthcare quality improvement. *BMJ,363*, k4907. https://doi.org/10.1136/bmj.k4907

Mate, G. (2018). *In the realm of hungry ghosts: Close encounters with addiction.* Vermillion.

Ministry of Health [Portugal]. (2000). *Decriminalisation: Portuguese legal framework applicable to the consumption of narcotics and psychotropic substances.* https://www.sicad.pt/BK/Dissuasao/Documents/Decriminalisation_Legislation.pdf

Mohankumar, R. (2022). *The influence of cultural stigma on perceptions of mental illness.* [Unpublished master's dissertation, San José State University].

Mongan, D., Millar, S. R., & Galvin, B. (2021). *The 2019–20 Irish national drug and alcohol survey: Main findings.* https://www.hrb.ie/fileadmin/2._Plugin_related_files/Publications/2021_publications/2021_HIE/Evidence_Centre/The_2019-20_Irish_National_Drug_and_Alcohol_Survey._Main_findings.pdf

Montagu, A. (1966). The long search for euphoria. *Reflections, 1,* 62–69.

Namou, W. (n.d.). History of merchants, beer in ancient Mesopotamia. *Chaldean News.* https://www.chaldeannews.com/features-1/2019/12/24/history-of-merchants-beer-in-ancient-mesopotamia

New South Wales Ministry of Health. (2015). *Evidence check review: Effective model of care for comorbid mental illness and illicit substance use.* https://www.health.nsw.gov.au/mentalhealth/resources/Publications/comorbid-mental-care-review.pdf

Norton, M. (2019). Implementing co-production in traditional, statutory mental health services. *Mental Health Practice, 27*(1). https://doi.org/10.7748/mhp.2019.e1304

Norton, M. J. (2022). *Co-production in mental health: Implementing policy into practice.* Routledge.

O'Halloran, M. (2018, February 15). Alcohol abuse costs Irish economy €2.3 billion a year, Dail hears. https://www.drugsandalcohol.ie/28583/#:~:text=Alcohol%20abuse%20costs%20Irish%20economy,bn%20a%20year%2C%20D%C3%A1il%20hears

O'Mahony, S. (2020). *A socio-historical deconstruction of the term "addiction" and an etiological model of drug addiction.* [Unpublished doctoral dissertation, University of Manchester].

Parker, C. B. (2014, July 16). Hallucinatory 'voices' shaped by local culture, Stanford anthropologist says. *Stanford News.* https://news.stanford.edu/2014/07/16/voices-culture-luhrmann-071614/

Pescosolido, B. A., Halpern-Manners, A., Luo, L., & Perry, B. (2021). Trends in public stigma of mental illness in the US, 1996–2018. *JAMA Network Open, 4*(12), e2140202. https://doi.org/10.1001/jamanetworkopen.2021.40202

Quigley, L. (2022). Gambling disorder and stigma: Opportunities for treatment and prevention. *Current Addiction Reports, 9,* 410–419. https://doi.org/10.1007/s40429-022-00437-4

Ross, C. A., & Margolis, R. L. (2018). Research domain criteria: Cutting edge neuroscience of Galen's humours revisited? *Molecular Neuropsychiatry, 4*(3), 158–163. https://doi.org/10.1159/000493685

Shi, H. D., McKee, S. A., & Cosgrove, K. P. (2022). Why language matters in alcohol research: Reducing stigma. *Alcohol: Clinical and Experimental Research, 46*(6), 1103–1109. https://doi.org/10.1111/acer.14840

Sinha, S. (2018, December 19). A visual journey through addiction. *The New York Times.* https://www.nytimes.com/interactive/2018/us/addiction-heroin-opioids.html

SMART Recovery. (2022). *Principles and positions.* https://smartrecovery.ie/about-us/

Subu, M. A., Wati, D. F., Netrida, N., Priscilla, V., Dias, J. M., Abraham, M. S., Slewa-Youinan, S., & Al-Yateem, N. (2021). Type of stigma experienced by patients with mental illness and mental health nurses in Indonesia: A qualitative content analysis. *International Journal of Mental Health Systems, 17,* 77. https://doi.org/10.1186/s13033-021-00502-x

Tarricone, J. (2020, September 10). *Richard Nixon and the origins of the war on drugs.* https://www.bostonpoliticalreview.org/post/richard-nixon-and-the-origins-of-the-war-on-drugs

Tasca, C., Rapetti, M., Carta, M. G., & Fadda, B. (2012). Women and hysteria in the history of mental health. *Clinical Practice and Epidemiology in Mental Health, 8,* 110–119. https://doi.org/10.2174/1745017901208010110

TD Consultancy. (n.d.). *History of cannabis/marijuana.* https://tonydagostino.co.uk/history-of-cannabis/

The Gateway Foundation. (2023, June 22). *Why doesn't punishment stop addiction.* https://www.gatewayfoundation.org/addiction-blog/why-does-punishment-not-stop-addiction/

United Nations. (1961). *Single convention on narcotic drugs, 1961.* https://www.unodc.org/pdf/convention_1961_en.pdf

United Nations. (1988). *United Nations convention against illicit traffic in narcotic drugs and psychotropic substances 1988.* https://www.unodc.org/pdf/convention_1988_en.pdf

We Change Laws. (n.d.). *Colorado and Washington: Life after legalization and regulation.* https://www.mpp.org/issues/legalization/colorado-and-washington-life-after-legalization-and-regulation/#:~:text=In%202012%2C%20Colorado%20and%20Washington,half%20of%20the%20U.S.%20population

Wisevoter. (2023). *Alcohol consumption by country.* https://wisevoter.com/country-rankings/alcohol-consumption-by-country/

World Health Organization. (2022, May 9). *Alcohol.* https://www.who.int/news-room/fact-sheets/detail/alcohol

Chapter 2

Mental Health, Addiction and Dual Diagnosis: National and International Policy Context

Oliver John Cullen[a] and Michael John Norton[b]

[a]*HSE Mental Health Services, Ireland*
[b]*HSE Office of Mental Health Engagement and Recovery, Ireland*

Abstract

The second chapter of this text provides an introduction to policy relating to mental health, addiction and dual diagnosis from three jurisdictions [Ireland, UK and Australia], chosen because of their close links to Irish people and mental health service provision. The chapter begins with an introduction, reflecting on key points raised in Chapter 1 and how they are relevant to this present chapter. A critical exploration of the policies within these three jurisdictional areas is then presented to highlight the strategic direction of mental health and addiction service provision within the three jurisdictions. This includes the acknowledgement that mental health and addiction services need to be integrated as the presence of dual diagnosis in modern society increases at an alarming rate. Finally, this chapter concludes with a link to each of the policies mentioned herein for those who wish to explore these issues further.

Keywords: Future healthcare; healthcare management; policy; recommendations; service delivery

Different Diagnoses, Similar Experiences:
Narratives of Mental Health, Addiction Recovery and Dual Diagnosis, 19–33
Copyright © 2024 by Oliver John Cullen and Michael John Norton
Published under exclusive licence by Emerald Publishing Limited
doi:10.1108/978-1-80455-848-520241002

2.1. Introduction

In the first chapter of this text, we explored the cultural perceptions as they relate to mental health and addiction. Here, we discovered that both were clouded and to some extent still are today in a fog of stigma, prejudice and misunderstanding. A large part of this relates to the legacy of mental ill health and addiction services since the beginning of the time, but more so in the last two to three hundred years. This current chapter adds to the context provided in Chapter 1 by exploring policy and how this has shaped services in three jurisdictions, chosen because of their tight links to Irish people and culture. Section 2.2 focuses on health policy within an Irish context. This includes a brief history of mental health and addiction policy before discussing in detail the current policy documents as they relate to mental health and addiction service delivery. Next, Section 2.3 explores similar policy contexts within the UK followed by Section 2.4 which explores policies within an Australian context. Finally, Section 2.5 concludes this narrative by summarising the key learnings from policy that impact mental health, addiction, and dual diagnosis service provision. Section 2.2 is now presented.

2.2. Health Policy in Ireland

Mental health policy within an Irish context is a relatively new feature within mental health discourse. Before 1984, there was no evidence of a policy for mental health in Ireland. There was, however, legislation that governed how mental health services should be run. Such legislation, like the Lunacy (Ireland) Act and the Lunacy Regulations (Ireland) Act, dated back over a century when those with mental health challenges were locked away in the old traditional asylums of the time, where modalities of treatment were often inhumane, barbaric and dehumanising (Chow & Priebe, 2013). Conditions here were eloquently described in Kilgannon's paper where entering the asylums was compared to '... *a decent into hell*' (Kilgannon, 2021).

In 1984, Ireland first released a mental health policy: '*The Psychiatric Services – Planning for the Future*', which aimed to transform service provision in line with emerging new sociological constructs such as human rights for those currently residing in asylums (Mann et al., 2016; Norton, 2019). The document was novel in the sense that it promised structural and cultural reform. However, the policy was set to ultimately fail due to the lack of traction from those on the grounds of mental health service provision (Norton, 2022).

Within addiction discourse, policy within an Irish context began in 2001, with the publication of '*Building on Experiences*' (Government of Ireland, 2001). The policy, which had a lifetime of seven years aimed to significantly reduce the harm caused by the misuse of drugs through supply reduction, prevention, treatment and research through a set of 100 individual actions (Government of Ireland, 2001). In 2009, after a review of the current policy at that time, a new strategy was produced (Department of Community, Rural and Gaeltacht Affairs, 2009).

This time through the Department of Community, Rural and Gaeltacht Affairs with the aim of continuing to tackle the harm caused by the misuse of drugs over another seven-year timeline. In this iteration, prevention and rehabilitation concepts were added to the previous domains identified in the '*Building on Experiences*' document.

Services continued to operate in the same way until the Department of Health created a modern iteration of the old policy, named: '*A Vision for Change*' (Norton, 2022). This policy set out a range of ideals to be completed within a 10-year period including the closure of the traditional asylums, the creation of community mental health teams, the embracement of personal recovery as an ideal that all services should strive towards and the implementation of lived experience workforce into traditional service provision. Although the above structural and cultural changes were made, the overall impact of the policy has been described as uneven at best with many of the promises made left incomplete (Mental Health Reform, 2017). Fig. 2.1 further illustrates the development of policy over time within an Irish context.

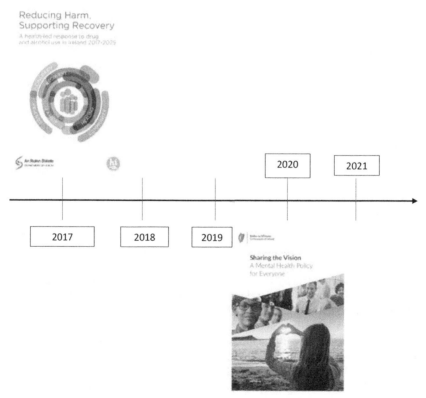

Fig. 2.1.   Irish Policy Timeline.

2.2.1. Reducing Harm, Supporting Recovery: 2017–2025

'*Reducing Harm, Supporting Recovery*' is an eight-year strategy co-produced by the Irish government and a variety of other stakeholders. It aimed to address the harm caused at a macro [societal], meso [community] and micro [person/family] level by illicit substances by 2025 (Department of Health, 2017). In order to achieve this, the strategy identified a vision that expressed a desire for:

> A healthier and safer Ireland, where public health and safety is protected and the harms caused to individuals, families and communities by substance misuse are reduced and every person affected by substance use is empowered to improve their health and wellbeing and quality of life. (Department of Health, 2017, p. 8)

This vision would be achieved by five SMART goals. The first goal was to **promote and protect health and wellbeing**. Here, the goal's objective is to support stakeholders in creating change that would reduce health inequities within our society. The idea which is that if these inequities are reduced, the early consumption of illicit substances, including alcohol, could be minimised and prevented (Department of Health, 2017). The second goal: **minimising the harm caused by the use and misuse of substances and promoting rehabilitation and recovery** outlines a four-tier person-centred model of support for those with a substance misuse difficulty.

Tier 1 documents basic information and advice. Tier 2 examines harm reduction supports inclusive of specialist addiction services. Tier 3 looks at specialist interventions in a range of settings. Finally, tier 4 documents specialised and dedicated inpatient and residential units necessary for the treatment of substance misuse disorders (Department of Health, 2017).

The third goal: **addressing the harms of drug markets and reducing access to drugs for harmful use**, looks at preventing such substances from ever reaching the drug markets on the streets. In addition, it seeks to tackle drug dealing and drug-related crime committed across the country through the availability of appropriate resources. The fourth goal within the strategy is to **support the participation of individuals, families and communities**. The strategy recognises the knowledge sets of all stakeholders involved in substance misuse, including the family unit and as such any local drug strategy should be co-produced with all relevant stakeholders. The final goal examines the **development of a sound and comprehensive evidence-informed policy and actions** so that there is an increased understanding between all stakeholders regarding substance misuse. Additionally, this also refers to creating an evidence base through the monitoring of a range of key performance indicators associated with the current strategy.

Although dual diagnosis is mentioned within this policy, it was not until the new model of care was developed that a referral pathway for those experiencing these phenomena was developed (Fig. 2.2).

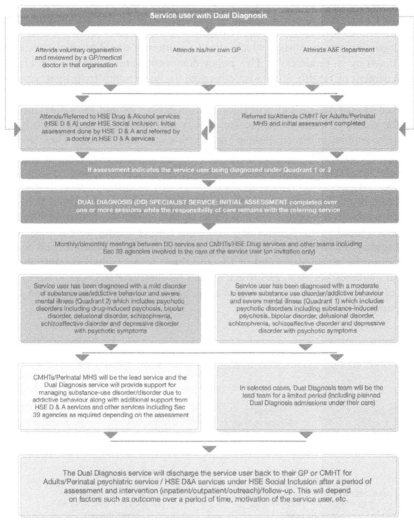

Fig. 2.2.   Referral Pathway for Dual Diagnosis.

In addition to the referral pathway, the new model of care also promotes the creation of specific dual diagnosis treatment teams consisting of a wide range of multidisciplinary stakeholders including members employed as a result of the work of the Mental Health Engagement and Recovery Office within the HSE (Health Service Executive, 2023). However, there is an acknowledgement from both the policy and the model of care that much more work is needed to attain these highly evidence-based standards (Department of Health, 2017; Health Service Executive, 2023).

2.2.2. Sharing the Vision: A Mental Health Policy for Everyone

In 2020, some 14 years after the release of '*A Vision for Change*', a new policy document was published which aimed to enhance the ideals and principles laid down by its predecessor. This policy document named '*Sharing the Vision*' (Department of Health, 2020) would become the latest policy to instigate change within service provision, particularly at the primary healthcare level. There are a number of core values and principles that underpin '*Sharing the Vision*' including the values of respect, compassion, equity and hope, followed by principles: recovery, trauma-informed, human rights and value and learning. These underpinning values and principles, help to inform each of the four domains on which the '*Sharing the Vision*' recommendations are based upon (Fig. 2.3).

The first domain: '*Promotion, Prevention and Early Intervention*' focuses on the promotion of mental health across the lifespan. Within this primary focus, comes mental health promotion in schools, so that students can identify stressors which can lead to mental ill health quicker, thereby preventing more serious mental distress from occurring. Additionally, the policy also discusses mental health promotion for those at the end of life and those with an intellectual disability. It also identifies key strategies which should be continued in order to maximise mental health promotion and stigma reduction, including '*Connecting for Life*' (Department of Health, 2015).

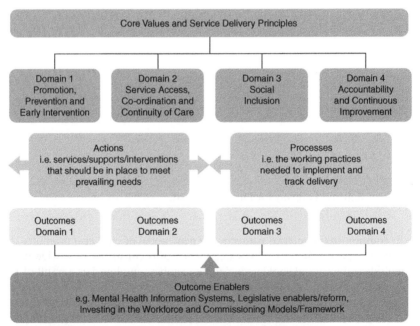

Fig. 2.3.   Organising Framework for Sharing the Vision. *Source*: Department of Health (2022) Implementation plan 2022–2024; Sharing the Vision. Sharing the Vision Implementation Team, Palmerstown Dublin.

The second domain: '*Service Access, Coordination and Continuity of Care*' sets out a tiered approach to mental health service provision in order to allow for timely evidence-based mental health interventions. Within this domain, it recognises the inability of services to cater for the diverse needs of those with mental health difficulties. Although there have been attempts in the past to develop a standardised approach that documents the service user journey from first referral to discharge, this pathway does not necessarily represent the journey in all mental health services today. As such, recommendation 39 of '*Sharing the Vision*' seeks to update this process map with the main elements that should be in a care pathway as documented.

In addition to care pathways, this domain of '*Sharing the Vision*' also examines the reconceptualisation of outpatient clinics as well as the power shift of removing psychiatry from the team lead role in order to create a more collaborative sharing of power amongst MDT team members. Finally, this domain also looks at initiatives that can prevent service users from entering the care pathway through initiatives like crisis cafés as well as peer-led interventions like Galway Community Café and Donegal's Peer Led Wellness Cafés. For those requiring services, '*Sharing the Vision*' promotes the move to telehealth as well as increasing the age of transfer from CAMHS to AMHS from 18 to 25 years.

'*Sharing the Vision*' recognises the overlap between mental illness and addiction, which when combined forms a dual diagnosis. In addition, it recognises that those with a dual diagnosis have the right to appropriate mental health service support in their recovery as those with mental health challenges alone. Unlike its predecessor, '*Sharing the Vision*' supports the integration of mental health and addiction services across both primary and secondary care, which is to be overseen by a national clinical programme and a model of care – which was published in mid-2023.

The third domain: '*Social Inclusion*' supports mental health and addiction service users to access housing, employment, education and training. These elements are also arising as important for recovery through the ideals of social recovery – which will be explored further in the next chapter – as stipulated by Norton and Swords (2020). This vision is to be achieved by the expansion of the Individualised Placement and Support [IPS] programme as well as the START project. The final domain: '*Accountability and Continuous Improvement*' aims to create a culture of accountability through a number of mechanisms including from service feedback by service users, family members/carers/supporters [recommendation 78] to the implementation of '*Slaintecare*' [recommendation 75] and adherence to other policies and standards like the Judgement Support Framework [recommendation 84].

2.3. Health Policy in the United Kingdom

Irish policy as it relates to health care closely follows that of the UK due to a number of factors including the proximity of the UK to Ireland, as well as the fact that up until approximately 100 years ago, Ireland was part of the commonwealth of the UK. Unlike, Australian policy [to follow], UK-based policy seems to be more reactive to the growing mental health and addiction crisis compared to other westernised countries. What follows is a critical discussion of UK policy as it relates to mental health and addiction services.

2.3.1. NHS Mental Health Implementation Plan 2019/20–2023/24

'*The NHS Mental Health Implementation Plan 2019/20–2023/24*' seeks to achieve a transformation of mental health services at its most ambitious level to date. This commitment was previously achieved by the '*Five Year Forward View for Mental Health.*' First published in 2016. This strategy was developed as a response to the change in public attitudes towards mental health services from one of paternalism to one of hope as service provision begins to embrace a recovery orientation. This is to be achieved by securing an additional £1 billion in funding, which will allow 1 million people to access the services by 2020/2021. The plan offers individuals a higher quality of care, whilst reducing stigma and promoting equal and positive relationships within communities. With the 2019/20–2023/24 plan, an additional £2.3 billion of funding was secured to provide high-quality client-centred care to approximately 370,000 adults across the mental health services (NHS Providers, 2019). The policy also examines the specific needs of specific populations such as:

1. Children and young people's mental health,
2. Adult severe mental illness community care,
3. Crisis and liaison services,
4. Suicide reduction and bereavement support,
5. Problem gambling mental health support,
6. Digital mental health and improving the quality of data.

(NHS Improvements, 2019)

2.3.2. From Harm to Hope: A 10-Year Drugs Plan to Cut Crime and Save Lives

'*From Harm to Hope*' documents a 10-year strategic plan agreed by the UK government to proactively and in some cases reactively combat the serious consequences of illicit substance misuse within UK society (Her Majesties Government, 2021). This is viewed by two separate prongs. The first examines reducing access to means by combatting the source of drugs in UK communities whilst the second prong highlights a system whereby one can recover and live a drug-free life. For the purposes of this book, we will only examine policy recommendations and promises related to this second prong.

Within UK health services, the strategic plan promises a world class treatment and recovery system, achieved through the allocation of an extra £780 million pounds over the lifetime of the strategy. These monies will be used to provide a wide variety of evidence-based supports that can support someone to move from active addiction to active recovery (Fig. 2.4) (Her Majesties Government, 2021).

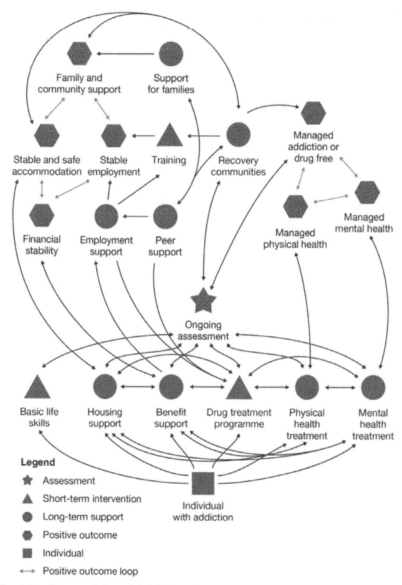

Fig. 2.4.   Systems Map of Addiction Supports.

In addition to this, the strategy promises to reduce stigma and save lives through a number of mechanisms including the better integration of services and improved employment opportunities for those in recovery from addiction (Her Majesties Government, 2021). This is in the hopes that by the end of the lifecycle of this policy, that the actions undertaken to adhere to the policy will have prevented up to 1,000 deaths in the UK whist increasing treatment capacity by 20% (Gov.UK, 2022).

2.4. Health Policy in Australia

The health policies in Australia unilaterally seek to use a more proactive approach to dealing with mental health and addiction challenges. The idea behind these policies is that when an individual is armed with appropriate information and a knowledge base early in their life and recovery journey, this can result in the promotion of recovery through de-stigmatisation and harm minimisation through a social and familial approach. This is achieved through partnership and collaboration with all stakeholders, including the more marginalised members of society. To further support discussions in relation to the major policies within an Australian context, see Fig. 2.5.

2.4.1. National Mental Health Policy 2008

The National Mental Health Policy 2008 – Australia seeks to implement a more recovery-orientated and collaborative approach to mental health structures and policies. Although some of the language in the policy may seem outdated in the context of 2023, we do see a stigma reduction approach that incorporates the individual and their lived experience, family and carers, clinical, education, community, housing and many other associated agencies thus capitalising on the participation and inclusion of a multi-faceted approach to recovery.

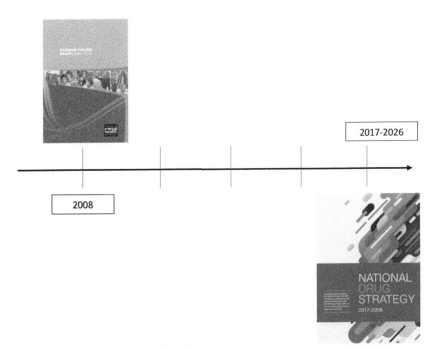

Fig. 2.5.   Australian Policy Timeline.

Australia is understood to be proactive in their approach to mental health recovery through continuous service development, policies, strategies and reports, seeking to explore more advantageous approaches to the challenges faced by individuals with enduring mental distress. Australia's National Mental Health Strategy was introduced in 1992 and compromised of:

- The National Mental Health Policy,
- The First National Mental Health Plan,
- The Mental Health Statement of Rights and Responsibilities,
- A funding agreement between the Commonwealth and the states and territories.

Fig. 2.6 documents the milestones in creating the National Mental Health Policy 2008.

The National Mental Health Policy 2008 gives acknowledgment to the unique contribution of the Indigenous communities, recognising their culture and their identity as a fundamental part of their own well-being (Commonwealth of Australia, 2009). The policy has a number of aims which include:

1. The promotion of mental health in the Australian community with the overall purpose of preventing mental health challenges from occurring.
2. Reducing the impact of mental health challenges, including stigma, on an individual, familial and community level.
3. The promotion of recovery from mental health challenges.
4. Upholding the rights of those who experience mental health challenges and enabling their meaningful participation in society.

The document describes an aspirational view of recovery that encompasses the mental health challenge itself and the empathetic, meaningful responses to the same that should be in place within service provision. The document also discusses dual diagnosis – termed here as 'comorbidity', with specific interest in regard to the symbiotic effects of mental health on addiction and vice versa (Commonwealth of Australia, 2009).

The policy further emphasises the rights and responsibilities of individuals who are challenged by mental health issues. It acknowledges the rights of individuals to live a life free of discrimination, with access to a range of applicable services that frame their recovery, also bearing in mind the responsibility of these individuals to work with the services for a better outcome. The individual's right to participate in their community must be upheld.

The complexity of mental health is multifaceted and involves a wide range of different agencies and partners, including accommodation, employment, community support, income and education (Fig. 2.7). Acknowledging the crucial role of family and carers, the policy highlights that those using services also require appropriate support from these stakeholders (Commonwealth of Australia, 2009).

This policy concludes that a positive outcome is achieved when the service, the individual and their family members/carers are all actively and meaningfully involved in the recovery process (Commonwealth of Australia, 2009).

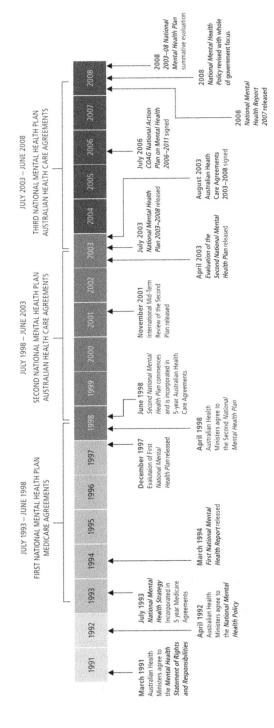

Note: COAG refers to Council of Australian Governments.

Fig. 2.6.   Milestones in the Development of the National Mental Health Strategy, 1991–2008. *Source:* ©Commonwealth of Australia 2009 as represented by the Department of Health and Aged Care.

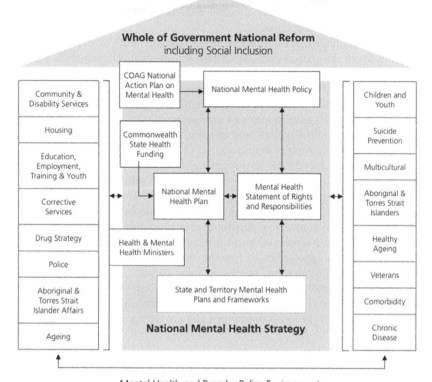

Fig. 2.7. Multiagency, Collaborate Approach to Mental Health Care.
Source: ©Commonwealth of Australia 2009 as represented by the Department of Health and Aged Care.

Additionally, the policy acknowledges the role of research in the journey towards recovery orientation, particularly, when this research is conducted in a way that honours the values of co-production as laid out by Norton (2022).

2.4.2. National Drug Strategy: 2017–2026

The '*National Drug Strategy: 2017–2026*' is reflective of previous policies published in Australia, by utilising the principles of previous policies to create a 10-year strategy that focuses on alcohol, tobacco and other drugs. It does this in the hope that various states will create accompanying action plans, that prioritise local issues. The policy outlines the rationale for such a strategy by providing examples of harm from drug use, from acute injuries to chronic conditions like hepatitis and HIV to economic harm on a micro [individual], meso [familial] and macro level [societal]. As a result, the strategy focuses on harm minimisation at these three levels of the social world, through being proactive rather than reactive. Examples of proactivity include demand reduction, harm minimisation, harm reduction and supply reduction.

The strategy describes a number of underpinning values of harm minimisation from which the actions discussed within are reflected. These include funding and resource allocation, which is dependent on current evidence-based practices. By constructing and sharing information, desired outcomes can be achieved. This is central to a harm minimisation approach. This sharing of knowledge creates partnerships between government and non-governmental agencies which is conducive to a joint, multi-departmental approach to supporting those with addiction, resulting in better use of resources.

The document also alludes to supporting individuals from cultural minorities within our society, particularly around the added sensitivities that may need to be observed to respect their ethnic minority status. This is imperative within the strategy due to the stigmatisation from elders and others within these ethnic communities, particularly in Australia, towards substance misuse (Bowen & Walton, 2015). The purpose of harm minimisation within this document is to use evidence-based approaches to improve outcomes. This document supports the aim of harm minimisation, keeping in mind cultural sensitivities, through a state-specific implementation plan. This will also allow for local accountability for initiatives related to the strategy through the monitoring of key performance indicators created by the local community, and not the national monitoring team.

2.5. Concluding Remarks

In summary, this chapter explored national and international policies as they relate to mental health, addiction and dual diagnosis. From a critical analysis of these policies, it can be concluded that these policies reflect a change in direction for both mental health and addiction services to a more person-centred, recovery-orientated service. Examples of this include the move towards co-production and collaborative working, where agency and stakeholders work together to achieve the best possible outcome for the end user and their families. This in turn will allow services to share the power between stakeholders, thereby reducing harm and governance concerns that follow. This issue of collaborative working will soon be discussed. However, before this occurs, the essence of recovery needs to be explored in these populations and as such is the subject of our next chapter of this text.

References

Bowen, E. A., & Walton, Q. L. (2015). Disparities and the social determinants of mental health and addictions: Opportunities for a multifaceted social work response. *Health & Social Work, 40*(3), e59–e65. https://doi.org/10.1093/hsw/hlv034

Chow, W. S., & Priebe, S. (2013). Understanding psychiatric institutionalisation: A conceptual review. *BMC Psychiatry, 13*, 169. https://doi.org/10.1186/1471-244X-13-169

Commonwealth of Australia. (2009). *National Mental Health Policy 2008*. https://www.health.gov.au/sites/default/files/documents/2020/11/national-mental-health-policy-2008.pdf

Department of Community, Rural and Gaeltacht Affairs. (2009). *National Drug Strategy Interim 2009–2016*. https://www.drugsandalcohol.ie/12388/1/DCRGA_Strategy_2009-2016.pdf

Department of Health. (2015). *Connecting for life: Ireland's national strategy to reduce suicide 2015–2020*. https://www.hse.ie/eng/services/list/4/mental-health-services/nosp/preventionstrategy/connectingforlife.pdf

Department of Health. (2017). *Reducing harm, supporting recovery: A health-led response to Drug and Alcohol use in Ireland 2017–2025*. http://www.drugs.ie/download-Docs/2017/ReducingHarmSupportingRecovery2017_2025.pdf

Department of Health. (2020). *Sharing the vision: A mental health policy for everyone*. https://www.gov.ie/pdf/?file=https://assets.gov.ie/76770/b142b216-f2ca-48e6-a551-79c208f1a247.pdf#page=null

Gov.UK. (2022). *Policy paper – from harm to hope: A 10 year drugs plan to cut crime and save lives*. https://www.gov.uk/government/publications/from-harm-to-hope-a-10-year-drugs-plan-to-cut-crime-and-save-lives/from-harm-to-hope-a-10-year-drugs-plan-to-cut-crime-and-save-lives#executive-summary

Government of Ireland. (2001). *Building on experience: National drug strategy 2001–2008*. https://www.drugsandalcohol.ie/5187/1/799-750.pdf

Health Service Executive. (2023). *Model of care for people with mental disorder and co-existing substance use disorder (dual diagnosis)*. https://www.hse.ie/eng/about/who/cspd/ncps/mental-health/dual-diagnosis-ncp/dual-diagnosis-model-of-care.pdf

Her Majesties Government. (2021). *From harm to hope: A 10 year drugs plan to cut crime and save lives*. https://assets.publishing.service.gov.uk/media/629078bad3bf7f036fc492d1/From_harm_to_hope_PDF.pdf

Kilgannon, D. (2021). A 'forgettable minority'? Psychiatric institutions and the intellectually disabled in Ireland, 1965–84. *Social History of Medicine, 34*(3), 808–827. https://doi.org/10.1093/shm/hkaa015

Mann, S. P., Bradley, V. J., & Sahakian, B. J. (2016). Human rights-based approaches to mental health. *Health and Human Rights Journal, 18*(1), 263–276.

Mental Health Reform. (2017). *Mental Health Reform submission on review of A Vision for Change*. https://www.mentalhealthreform.ie/wp-content/uploads/2017/09/Submission-on-review-of-A-Vision-for-Change.pdf

NHS Improvements. (2019). *NHS mental health implementation plan 2019/20–2023/24*. https://www.longtermplan.nhs.uk/wp-content/uploads/2019/07/nhs-mental-health-implementation-plan-2019-20-2023-24.pdf

NHS Providers. (2019). *NHS mental health implementation plan 2019/20 – 2023/24*. https://nhsproviders.org/media/688000/nhs-mental-health-implementation-plan-2019-briefing-010819.pdf

Norton, M. (2019). Implementing co-production in traditional statutory mental health services. *Mental Health Practice, 27*(1). https://doi.org/10.7748/mhp.2019.e1304

Norton, M. J. (2022). *Co-Production in mental health: Implementing policy into practice*. Routledge.

Norton, M. J., & Swords, C. (2020). Social recovery: A new interpretation to recovery-orientated services – A critical literature review. *The Journal of Mental Health Training, Education and Practice, 16*(1), 7–20. https://doi.org/10.1108/JMHTEP-06-2020-0035

Chapter 3

Recovery in Mental Health, Addiction and Dual Diagnosis

Michael John Norton[a] and Oliver John Cullen[b]

[a]HSE Office of Mental Health Engagement and Recovery, Ireland
[b]HSE Mental Health Services, Ireland

Abstract

The term recovery is an abstract concept. It differs for each and every person regardless of race, sexual orientation, culture or belief system. Throughout the age of modern medicine, doctors and scholars have tried to understand the concept of recovery for those in mental distress and those who are in the process of addiction. This chapter aims to highlight the different understandings of the concept of recovery from both a mental health and addiction perspective in order to gain a more in-depth understanding of the processes of recovery and how its definition and qualities have changed over time as new and more compelling clinical evidence emerges.

Keywords: Biomedicine; mental health; personal journey; recovery; social world

3.1. Introduction

Chapter 3 aims to demonstrate the position of traditional clinical services as a response to the treatment of mental ill health and addiction. Section 3.2 documents the clinical response to mental ill health as a '*reduction of symptoms*' with the aid of medications and clinical interventions to address the imbalances within the brain of the individual. It gives rise to a '*one size fits all*' position, that can lead to poor outcomes for the individual. This chapter discusses the civil rights movement that focuses on the personal nuances of the individual and the need for a

Different Diagnoses, Similar Experiences:
Narratives of Mental Health, Addiction Recovery and Dual Diagnosis, 35–41
Copyright © 2024 by Michael John Norton and Oliver John Cullen
Published under exclusive licence by Emerald Publishing Limited
doi:10.1108/978-1-80455-848-520241003

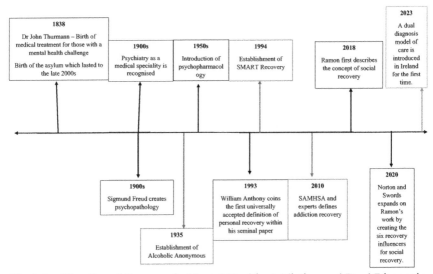

Fig. 3.1.   Timeline of Recovery in Mental Health, Addiction and Dual Diagnosis.

more personal approach to recovery. This approach offers personal responsibility to the individual and their own care. Within the text, one can see the by-product of family recovery as its own journey, and the role that the wider community plays in embracing the opportunities that are now available in supporting individuals on a wider scale. Section 3.3 documents the personal responsibilities of the person in addiction. It outlines the isolative effect of the disorder, and how connection can re-establish the person's sense of identity. This is achieved through a deeper understanding through peer support at a practical level such as the '*12 step model*'. The chapter here shows real evidence of the recovery community healing within itself and echoing out into the wider community. For a brief synopsis of what is covered in this chapter, please refer to Fig. 3.1. Finally, Section 3.4 concludes this chapter. Section 3.2 will now be discussed.

3.2. Recovery in Mental Health

Since the time of Dr John Thurman, a biomedical understanding of recovery has been promoted and endorsed by evidence-based medicine (Dickinson, 1990). It is a process which involves the eradication of signs and symptoms of mental distress. Such signs and symptoms arise from psychopathology incorporating either a chemical imbalance of neurotransmitters or physical structural abnormality within the brain itself. McDaid (2013) calls this understanding of mental distress and recovery: clinical recovery. In her 2013 technical report, she states that recovery clinically involves:

> an individual's mental state at a point in time, as measured by a clinician using standard criteria. Clinical recovery generally refers to a reduction in ... symptoms of a mental health condition.

> It can be measured by assessing the extent to which an individual
> still meets a diagnosis for a mental disorder or the extent to which
> their psychosocial functioning fits in with standardised norms.
> (McDaid, 2013)

Such measurements are often quantitative in nature and involve the use of diagnostic manuals such as the '*Diagnostic and Statistical Manual for Mental Disorders*' and/or the '*International Classification of Diseases*'. Despite the use of a positivist position, it is difficult to measure recovery in individuals using this paradigm as recovery is different for each individual and what works for one, may not work for another – making the concept even more difficult to quantify or justify through positivist means alone.

Unlike, clinical recovery, personal recovery originated from the civil rights movement in the 1980s and 1990s and as such is defined differently depending on personal factors, the context where recovery is being sought and the social world that surrounds the individual (Cook et al., 2017; Davidson et al., 2021). Within a mental health context, there are many different definitions of recovery as it is a personal and unique process (Ballesteros-Urpi et al., 2019; Piat et al., 2009). However, personal recovery is best described by the seminal work of William Anthony who suggests that recovery is:

> a deeply personal unique process of changing one's attitudes, values, feelings, goals, skills and/or roles. It is a way of living a satisfying hopeful and contributing life even with the limitations caused by illness... includes the development of new meaning and purpose in life as one grows beyond the catastrophic effects of mental illness. (Anthony, 1993, p. 21)

From this definition, one can see that recovery is not something that professionals do to service users, rather it is a personal process that is self-defined by the individual as they embark on their recovery journey (Watts & Higgins, 2017). In addition, personal recovery is described as a lifelong journey of discovery which is non-linear in orientation (Erondu & McGraw, 2021). However, despite the fact that the process is unique and different to each individual, Leamy et al. (2011) have highlighted five key ingredients necessary for recovery to occur. These key ingredients are explained through the acronym CHIME: **C**onnectiveness, **H**ope, **I**dentity, **M**eaning and Purpose, and **E**mpowerment (Leamy et al., 2011). Put simply, recovery can be described as '*someone to love, somewhere to live and something to do*' (Swords & Norton, 2023a). In today's mental health services, personal recovery is the ideal for many individuals and as such, this typology of recovery is still reflected today as a cornerstone in mental health policy and practice within service provision (Swords & Norton, 2023b).

Another facet that came as a by-product of the personal recovery movement is that of family recovery. This was conceptualised as a result of the recognition that family members also have a recovery journey to follow resulting from their loved one's use of the services (Cuskelly et al., 2022). For the purposes of this text, the

Health Service Executive's definition of family recovery will be used. Here, family recovery is described as:

> [...] intrinsically about all members of the family being able to live a life of their own choosing regardless of the challenges of mental health issues...respecting and accepting that while we all see things differently there are key skills we can draw on to live a life with hope, empathy, equality and autonomy. (Health Service Executive, 2018)

Despite resulting as a byproduct of the personal recovery movement, the evidence base for the concept is growing through the work of multiple scholars like those involved in the **PRIMERA** family project at Maynooth University, Ireland and through the first author's work in exploring enablers to family recovery (Cuskelly et al., 2022; Furlong et al., 2021a, 2021b; Norton & Cuskelly, 2021).

The process of recovery is everchanging as one discovers what is meaningful in their lives and what constructs recovery for them. Recently, our understanding of recovery has further evolved to assimilate the impact that the wider community plays in supporting an individual's recovery. This type of recovery began with Ramon (2018) who suggests that recovery is a:

> [...] journey of people experiencing mental ill health towards regaining social recognition and acceptance, in the form of their social identity or presence. (Ramon, 2018)

In other words, social recovery defined by Ramon and later by Norton and Swords (2020) suggests that recovery is socially constructed by members of society. It involves the factors needed for one to become part of and contribute to one's society again. Examples of which include housing and support (Norton & Swords, 2020). Although at the time of writing, there are three confirmed definitions of recovery, this is bound to expand as our empirical understanding of the concept deepens further. We now present how recovery can be contextualised differently through Section 3.3 which examines the concept of recovery but from within an addiction space.

3.3. Recovery in Addiction

Addiction recovery is a multifaceted, deeply personal journey for the individual. It shares similarities between peers that create a unique bonding experience, through emotional and empathetic understanding. Whilst addiction can create an isolative effect, this is further transpired through damaging personal relationships between family members, friends and one's own community. It is these peer connections within recovery circles that create healing. This relationship can often give the individual an opportunity to glance at and truly grasp a more recovery-orientated lifestyle (Alcoholic Anonymous, 2023). In 1935, Alcoholic

Anonymous (AA) created a template that would help individuals seek an understanding of recovery and realise its long-term potential through a 12-step model that has been empirically proven to change people's lives for nearly a century. With the growing nature of substance misuse, branches of AA were created to respond to these needs. For example, Narcotics Anonymous (NA), Cocaine Anonymous (CA) and Al-Anon Family Groups and Gambling Anonymous (GA). Founded in 1994 SMART Recovery (SMART Recovery, n.d.) was developed as a secular recovery option based on scientific evidence and the use of cognitive behavioural therapy (CBT).

With modern recovery, we understand that the traditional approach still holds weight for many individuals. Examples include inpatient treatment, detox with access to clinical care and recovery supports and outpatient treatment. In 2010, the Substance Abuse and Mental Health Services Administration (SAMHSA) (SAMHSA, 2012) along with leading experts in the field defined addiction recovery as:

> A process of change through which individuals improve their health and wellness, live a self- directed life, and strive to reach their full potential. (SAMHSA, 2012, p. 3)

This definition outlines a change that is evident in practice today. The description demonstrates personal responsibility for an individual in recovery. SAMHSA describes this through 10 Guiding Principles of Recovery: hope; person-driven; many pathways; holistic; peer support; relational; culture; addresses trauma; strengths/responsibility; and respect, whilst also delineating that there are four major factors to a life in recovery: Health, Home, Purpose and Community (SAMHSA, 2012).

3.4. Conclusion

Chapter 3 discusses recovery from both mental health and addiction. It closely examines the more recent historical changes within these movements and reflects on the changing attitudes towards said challenges within the confines of these struggles. We see a shift towards a less stigmatising approach and a more informed and inclusive community approach where individuals now understand that there are many different solutions to the challenges faced by the individual. We see themes in the text that echo recovery from a non-clinical perspective, such as peer support, hope, and personal reflection. The text shows the need for a multi-faceted approach to recovery that gives rise to individuals being self-driven on their own personal journeys of recovery. Finally, we see the need for the clinical approach to complement the timing of handing back the personal responsibility to the individual giving a more person-centred approach to their own care. In Chapter 4, we will explore mental health and addiction as co-occurring disorders and the model of care that best complements these conditions.

References

Alcoholic Anonymous. (2023). *History of A.A.* https://www.aa.org/aa-history

Anthony, W. A. (1993). Recovery from mental illness: The guiding vision of the mental health system in the 1990s. *Psychosocial Rehabilitation Journal, 16*(4), 11–23. https://psycnet.apa.org/doi/10.1037/h0095655

Ballesteros-Urpi, A., Slade, M., Manley, D., & Pardo-Hernandez, H. (2019). Conceptual framework for personal recovery in mental health among children and adolescents: A systematic review and narrative synthesis protocol. *BMJ Open, 9*(8), e029300. https://doi.org/10.1136/bmjopen-2019-029300

Cook, J., Morrow, M., & Battersby, L. (2017). Intersectional policy analysis of self-directed mental health care in Canada. *Psychiatric Rehabilitation Journal, 40*(2), 244–251. https://doi.org/10.1037/prj0000266

Cuskelly, K., Norton, M. J., & Delaney, G. (2022). Examining the existing knowledge base for enablers of family recovery in mental health: A protocol for a scoping review of national and international literature. *BMJ Open, 12*, e066484. https://doi.org/10.1136/bmjopen-2022-066484

Davidson, L., Rowe, M., DiLeo, P., Bellamy, C., & Delphin-Rittmon, M. (2021). Recovery-orientated systems of care: A perspective on the past, present and future. *Alcohol Research, 41*(1), 9. https://doi.org/10.35946/arcr.v41.1.09

Dickinson, E. (1990). From madness to mental health: A brief history of psychiatric treatments in the UK from 1800 to the present. *British Journal of Occupational Therapy, 53*(10), 419–424.

Erondu, C., & McGraw, C. (2021). Exploring the barriers and enablers to the implementation and adoption of recovery-orientated practice by community mental health provider organisations in England. *Social Work in Mental Health, 19*(5), 457–475. https://doi.org/10.1080/15332985.2021.1949426

Furlong, M., McGilloway, S., Mulligan, C., Killion, M. G., McGarr, S., Grant, A., Davidson, G., & Donaghy, M. (2021a). COVID-19 and families with parental mental illness: Crisis and opportunity. *Frontiers in Psychiatry, 12*, 567447.https://doi.org/10.3389/fpsyt.2021.567447

Furlong, M., McGilloway, S., Mulligan, C., McGuinness, C., & Whelan, N. (2021b). Family talk versus usual services in improving child and family psychosocial functioning in families with parental mental illness (PRIMERA – promoting research and innovation in mental hEalth seRvices for fAmilies and children): Study protocol for a randomised controlled trial. *Trials, 22*(1), 243. https://doi.org/10.1186/s13063-021-05199-4

Health Service Executive. (2018). *Family recovery guidance document 2018–2020: Supporting 'A national framework for recovery in mental health 2018–2020.* https://www.hse.ie/eng/services/list/4/mental-health-services/advancingrecoveryireland/national-framework-for-recovery-in-mental-health/family-recovery-guidance-document-2018-to-2020.pdf

Leamy, M., Bird, V., Le Boutillier, C., Williams, J., & Slade, M. (2011). Conceptual framework for personal recovery in mental health: Systematic review and narrative synthesis. *The British Journal of Psychiatry, 199*(6), 445–452. https://doi.org/10.1192/bjp.bp.110.083733

McDaid, S. (2013). Recovery …*what you should expect from a good quality mental health service.* https://www.mentalhealthreform.ie/wp-content/uploads/2013/03/MHR-Recovery-paper-final-April-2013.pdf

Norton, M. J., & Cuskelly, K. (2021). Family recovery interventions with families of mental health service users: A systematic review of the literature. *International Journal of Environmental Research and Public Health, 18*(15), 7858. https://doi.org/10.3390/ijerph18157858

Norton, M. J., & Swords, C. (2020). Social recovery: A new interpretation to recovery-orientated services – A critical literature review. *The Journal of Mental Health Training, Education and Practice, 16*(1), 7–20. https://doi.org/10.1108/JMHTEP-06-2020-0035

Piat, M., Sabetti, J., Couture, A., Sylvestre, J., Provencher, H., Botschner, J., & Stayner, D. (2009). What does recovery mean to me? Perspectives of Canadian mental health consumers. *Psychiatric Rehabilitation Journal, 32*(3), 199–207. https://doi.org/10.2975/32.3.2009.199.207

Ramon, S. (2018). The place of social recovery in mental health and related services. *International Journal of Environmental Research and Public Health, 15*(6), 1052. https://doi.org/10.3390/ijerph1506105

SAMHSA. (2012). *SAMHSA's Working definition of recovery.* https://store.samhsa.gov/sites/default/files/pep12-recdef.pdf

SMART Recovery. (n.d.). Our impact. https://www.smartrecoveryinternational.org/our-impact#:~:text=History%20of%20SMART%20Recovery,12%2DStep%20addiction%20recovery%20program

Swords, C., & Norton, M. J. (2023a). *What does recovery really mean in mental health today.* https://www.rte.ie/brainstorm/2023/0912/1404876-what-does-recovery-really-mean-in-mental-health-today/

Swords, C., & Norton, M. J. (2023b). Individual recovery or collective recovery? Do we really consider both in current Irish mental health policy and provision. *Irish Journal of Psychological Medicine,* 1–2. https://doi.org/10.1017/ipm.2023.25

Watts, M., & Higgins, A. (2017). *Narratives of recovery from mental illness: The role of peer support.* Routledge.

Chapter 4

The Conundrum of Dual Diagnosis

Oliver John Cullen

HSE Mental Health Services, Ireland

Abstract

Dual diagnosis [co-occurring mental health and addiction challenges] and recovery from the same are multifaceted and complex issues. These multifaceted and complex issues are difficult, time-consuming and require a multi-agency approach to their treatment. This chapter aims to present the characteristics that embody co-occurring disorders with the idea of defining this symbiotic relationship for the reader. This text will also highlight the paucity of resources currently available to those with a dual diagnosis.

Keywords: Dual diagnosis; addiction; mental health; co-occurring disorders; co-morbidity; recovery

4.1. Introduction

Until June 2020, when '*Sharing the Vision*' was first published, the separation of mental health and addiction as two separate entities that do not intertwine has created divergent understandings of recovery, which has inadvertently created systemic barriers to dual diagnosis recovery (Cullen & Norton, 2021; Kelly & Holahan, 2022; Swords & Norton, 2020). Chapter 4 examines the conundrum that is dual diagnosis as it relates to both the mental health and addiction space and views them together as co-occurring disorders. This chapter will discuss the nuances of dual diagnosis and the barriers for the individual as they seek a pathway to recovery from both challenges. The chapter aims to do this through Section 4.2, which will examine the current challenges of dual

Different Diagnoses, Similar Experiences:
Narratives of Mental Health, Addiction Recovery and Dual Diagnosis, 43–46
Copyright © 2024 by Oliver John Cullen
Published under exclusive licence by Emerald Publishing Limited
doi:10.1108/978-1-80455-848-520241004

diagnosis on both mental health and addiction discourse. This is then followed by Section 4.3 which concludes this chapter by highlighting the key learnings gained through such exploration conducted as part of Section 4.2. Section 4.2 is now presented.

4.2. Current Challenges to Mental Health and Addiction Discourse

Dual diagnosis can be simply defined as two co-occurring disorders (Cullen & Norton, 2021). However, empirically, there is no consensus regarding this terminology (Black, 2021). Despite this, although, two co-occurring disorders could mean different things to different people, for the purposes of this text, we stipulate that these co-occurring disorders originate from both a mental health and addiction challenge. Mental health and addiction challenges are often observed to occur in tandem with each other. In fact, almost 30% of those with a mental health challenge will also have a co-occurring substance use disorder at some point in their lives (Corace et al., 2022). A rationale for this is that the individual in question can make poor life decisions that may be based on their current perspective of life due to a mental health challenge and can utilise illicit substances in an effort to self soothe or block the pain that is present due to either the acute or chronic nature of the said challenge.

Today, there is much debate about what comes first, the mental health challenge or the addiction (Cullen & Norton, 2021; Richert et al., 2020). Additionally, there is a paucity of research as it pertains to the prevention and treatment of such co-occurring disorders (Baingana et al., 2015). However, research has suggested that up to half of individuals attending community mental health services struggle with substance misuse (Health Service Executive, 2023). Despite such awareness of the intertwined nature of these issues, it's only in more recent times that one can see a greater push towards treating both issues concurrently. As outlined in 'Sharing the Vision' recognition is given to the occurrence of these challenges and the right to access these health supports at the primary care level. Recommendations from the document suggest a multi-disciplinary approach including addiction counsellors to fully support the recovery process in getting the individual with co-occurring disorders the best possible outcome from the service (Department of Health, 2020).

Through public consultation, and the concerns raised regarding dual diagnosis, 'Reducing Harm, Supporting Recovery, A Health Led Response to Drug and Alcohol Use in Ireland 2017–2025' was created to stress the need for access to appropriate treatment and timely referral processes (Department of Health, 2017). The strategy discusses, for the first time in Irish health literature, the development of the dual diagnosis clinical programme, which aims to adopt an evidence-based approach to the identification of those with a dual diagnosis and the appropriate therapeutic approach to follow when treating an individual with a mental health and co-occurring substance misuse issue in order to improve recovery outcomes (Department of Health, 2017).

Currently, in Ireland, there are a number of in-treatment facilities that accommodate the treatment of those with a dual diagnosis: St John of God Hospital,[1] Smarmore Castle[2] and St Patricks Mental Health Services.[3] Each of these facilities offers a dual care system that helps individuals navigate through their challenges with expert care teams available throughout the process. Despite the fact that there are three services dedicated to the treatment of dual diagnosis in Ireland, they are all privately run which effectively puts a paywall between those needing treatment and the most appropriate services for them. This is even more damming when we consider the treatment of dual diagnosis in public services. Although public services have gone a long way in ensuring the appropriate structures are readily available for service use, there is still no official line of treatment in place.

Addiction, like mental health, is a complex, socioeconomic issue and the co-occurrence of both is well documented throughout history, ever since it was first identified within the literature in the 1980s (Hryb et al., 2007). But without treatment for both, together in tandem, there are multiple complexities including: the exasperation of symptoms and the over-reliance on substances to dampen down the psychological pain imposed by mental health challenges or compounded trauma that a person may experience. For example, veterans of the Vietnam War were subsequently diagnosed with post-traumatic stress disorder [PTSD] after admission to a chemical dependency unit (Hyer et al., 1991).

In their article: '*Dual Diagnosis in a Forensic Patient Sample: A Preliminary Tripartite Investigation to Inform Group Treatment Delivery for Substance Use*' Krishnan and Ireland (2023) found that two-thirds [8] of their participants described using substances to alleviate symptoms of mental health challenges. Stigma and its negative effects are still evident today across many cultures and systems, but with time, our perspectives on these conditions have changed. Behind the substance abuse, we now know lies a deeper traumatised self who is struggling to deal with intense psychological emotions resulting in the misuse of substances to dull the pain and survive another day in hell.

4.3. Conclusion

In summary, this chapter examined mental ill health and addiction as co-occurring disorders. When observing treatment solutions for the end user, the options are somewhat limited. The Department of Health and related services are responding to the crisis, but unfortunately not fast enough. With a myriad of compounded issues that surround dual diagnosis as a health condition, individuals, families, communities and services are at the mercy of the pace of this response. Whilst information is more readily available than ever before, the crisis

---

[1]https://stjohnofgodhospital.ie/
[2]https://www.smarmore-rehab-clinic.com/
[3]https://www.stpatricks.ie/

and the interventions required need to be further studied in order to provide an evidence-based response as promised within the new Model of Care for dual diagnosis.

References

Baingana, F., al'Absi, M., Becker, A. E., & Pringle, B. (2015). Global research challenges and opportunities for mental health and substance-use disorders. *Nature, 527*(7578), S172–S177. https://doi.org/10.1038/nature16032

Black, L.-A. (2021). *Mental ill health and substance misuse: Dual diagnosis.* http://www.niassembly.gov.uk/globalassets/documents/raise/publications/2017-2022/2021/health/1921.pdf

Corace, K., Ares, I., Overington, L., & Kim, H. S. (2022). Substance use and mental health disorders: Psychologists role in bridging the gap. *Canadian Psychology, 63*(3), 405–412. https://doi.org/10.1037/cap0000299

Cullen, O. J., & Norton, M. J. (2021). Chicken or egg: A dual diagnosis narrative. *Journal of Psychiatric and Mental Health Nursing, 29*(4), 507–511. https://doi.org/10.1111/jpm.12801

Department of Health. (2017). Reducing *harm, supporting recovery*: A health-led response to drug and alcohol use in Ireland 2017–2025. http://www.drugs.ie/download-Docs/2017/ReducingHarmSupportingRecovery2017_2025.pdf

Department of Health. (2020). *Sharing the VISION: A mental health policy for everyone.* https://assets.gov.ie/76770/b142b216-f2ca-48e6-a551-79c208f1a247.pdf

Health Service Executive. (2023). Dual diagnosis. https://www.hse.ie/eng/about/who/cspd/ncps/mental-health/dual-diagnosis-ncp/

Hryb, K., Kirkhart, R., & Talbert, R. (2007). A call for standardized definition of dual diagnosis. *Psychiatry, 4*(9), 15–16.

Hyer, L., Leach, P., Boudewyns, P. A., & Davis, H. (1991). Hidden PTSD in substance abuse inpatients among Vietnam veterans. *Journal of Substance Abuse Treatment, 8*(4), 213–219. https://doi.org/10.1016/0740-5472(91)90041-8

Kelly, K., & Holahan, R. (2022). *Dual recovery:A qualitative exploration of the views of stakeholders working in mental health, substance use and homelessness in Ireland on the barriers to recovery for individuals with a dual diagnosis.* https://mentalhealthreform.ie/wp-content/uploads/2022/05/Dual-Recovery-Full-Report.pdf

Krishnan, N., & Ireland, J. L. (2023). Dual diagnosis in a forensic patient sample: A preliminary tripartite investigation to inform group treatment delivery for substance use. *Journal of Forensic Psychology Research and Practice*, 1–36. https://doi.org/10.1080/24732850.2023.2281431

Richert, T., Anderberg, M., & Dahlberg, M. (2020). Mental health problems among young people in substance use treatment in Sweden. *Substance Abuse Treatment, Prevention, and Policy, 15*, 43. https://doi.org/10.1186/s13011-020-00282-6

Swords, C., & Norton, M. J. (2020). Is sharing really caring? A vision or an aspiration? Ireland's new mental health policy 2020. *Irish Journal of Psychological Medicine, 40*(2), 310–311. https://doi.org/10.1017/ipm.2020.118

Chapter 5

Co-production and the Lived Experience Perspective

Michael John Norton

HSE Office of Mental Health Engagement and Recovery, Ireland

Abstract

User involvement and co-production are imperative to the design, delivery and evaluation of service provision. This chapter provides a brief introduction to these concepts as they relate to mental health, addiction and dual diagnosis. This occurs through an exploration of models of user involvement, particularly, Arnstein's ladder of participation and MHERs engagement continuum. This is followed by exploring the benefits of user involvement at both a micro and macro level. Co-production – as the highest form of participation is also introduced followed by how these concepts are noted within policy. These concepts are imperative to the creation of a recovery-orientated service that meets the needs of the whole person and their supporters.

Keywords: Co-production; user involvement; recovery; policy; engagement

5.1. Introduction

Engagement is a term used to describe how service providers work together with service users and their support networks to actively involve them in decisions regarding service design, delivery, evaluation and policy (Health Service Executive, 2023c). Within this space, the term can be used interchangeably with words like participation and involvement (Cooper et al., 2023). However, for this chapter, user involvement will be used as the overall term. In recent years,

Different Diagnoses, Similar Experiences:
Narratives of Mental Health, Addiction Recovery and Dual Diagnosis, 47–55
Copyright © 2024 by Michael John Norton
Published under exclusive licence by Emerald Publishing Limited
doi:10.1108/978-1-80455-848-520241005

user involvement has been promoted at all levels of the service to improve the quality of the health service received by those who require them (Omeni et al., 2014). One reason for this is its documented benefits in every facet of service provision, including within service development (Kujala, 2008). The aim of this chapter is to introduce, you, the reader, to the concept of user involvement as this is the future of healthcare both in Ireland and internationally. This exploration will begin with Section 5.2 which will examine models of user involvement within both the peer-reviewed and grey literature. This is followed by Section 5.3, which explores user involvement's relationship with recovery. This leads us to Section 5.4, where co-production is discussed. Again, Section 5.5 will expand on Section 5.4 by relating user involvement to relevant policy contexts. Section 5.6 will then conclude the chapter. An overview of the models of user involvement will now be presented.

5.2. Models of User Involvement

There have been advancements in the conceptualisation and operationalisation of user involvement in health service provision and research in recent years (Tierney et al., 2014). This is particularly the case when it comes to the various models used to theorise user involvement within health discourse. Each model utilises a ladder to symbolise the various levels of user involvement in health care. The first model was developed by Sherry Arnstein in the 1960s (Fig. 5.1).

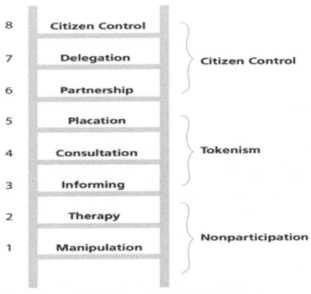

Fig. 5.1.   Sherry Arnstein's Ladder of Citizen Participation.

This ladder of participation illustrates various levels of participation through eight rungs divided into three broad categories: nonparticipation, tokenism and citizen control (Norton, 2022). At the bottom of the ladder lies the category of nonparticipation which is home to the rungs of manipulation and therapy. Here Arnstein (1969) suggests that there is no participation of the user. Instead, tasks are carried out by the person, with the person being the passive recipient of care (Norton, 2021). The middle category, entitled tokenism is home to the rungs: informing, consultation, and placation (Arnstein, 1969). Within these rungs form types of participation which is the minimum one can give in order to state that they are inclusive of other stakeholders in the act of participation. Finally, the last set of rungs: partnership, delegation and citizen control form part of the category citizen control. Here, participation ranges from being involved, to as an equal and finally to a revolution where service users are now doing to service providers rather than vice versa.

Since 1969, this ladder has undergone several amendments and iterations (Norton, 2021, 2022). The latest version of the ladder comes from the Office of Mental Health Engagement and Recovery, which forms part of the Health Service Executive's mental health services in their strategy: '*Engaged in Recovery*' (Health Service Executive, 2023a). Within this, a complete change in the wording of the ladder is proposed, but little has changed in terms of the positionality of the rungs or their intended meaning (Fig. 5.2).

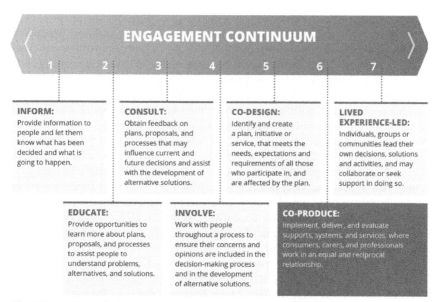

Fig. 5.2.   MHER's Engagement Continuum. *Source*: MHER Engagement Framework (2024).

5.3. User Involvement and the Recovery Journey

When examining user involvement within the literature, a prominent feature is the challenges of obtaining full, authentic involvement of users, with little attention paid to the benefits of this endeavour (Brown & Jones, 2021; Lawn, 2015). In order to support a more balanced conversation of this topic in the literature, the current chapter will now focus on the benefits of user involvement within mental health discourse from both the user and organisational perspectives.

5.3.1. Benefits of User Involvement to the Person

In terms of benefits to the user, Aase et al. (2021) categorise them into three main broad headings: legitimacy, access and insight. Legitimacy in this case refers to the acceptability of lived experience as a unique and equal knowledge set to that of learned knowledge. The key to user involvement at any level is the recognition that service users are experts on themselves and their unique circumstances due to their lived experiences of mental health difficulty (Tait & Lester, 2005). This is slowly occurring within behavioural services through the employment of peer-based roles such as Peer Support Workers. The idea behind such roles is that the peer utilises their lived experience to support others in recovery. In this sense, the lived experience transforms into a knowledge set that is on par with learned knowledge and when utilised correctly, it can increase the quality of the service (Norton, 2023). There is sparse research on this area of study currently as it is only within the past number of years that the knowledge set created by lived experiences: experiential knowledge has been realised as having therapeutic value.

In terms of access, there are a number of mechanisms available depending on the rationale for user involvement. If one looks at user involvement from an Irish context, its use for therapeutic processes would have begun in the early 2010s with a Genio-funded project to introduce the first Peer Support Workers into services. This project was deemed successful and in 2015, Naughton and colleagues released a position paper examining how Peer Support Workers can be integrated into traditional mental health systems (Naughton et al., 2015). In 2017, this would come to fruition and currently, at the time of writing, there were 28 Peer Support Workers employed by the health services in Ireland (Hunt & Byrne, 2019). Consequently, in 2015, Genio also funded the establishment of a family peer support service: Bealach Nua, which provides peer support services to family members of loved ones with a mental health challenge (Connaught Telegraph, 2020; Health Service Executive, 2023b). In 2021, this service was too brought in as part of the statutory health services with eleven family peers now *in situ* across the island of Ireland.

Since 2014, these lived experience perspectives were further cemented as imperative to all aspects of mental health service processes through the establishment of the first recovery college: Mayo Recovery College. Recovery colleges/education services focus on learning rather than cure and in doing so transform an individual from a passive patient to someone who is empowered to live life, despite the vulnerabilities they may experience due to a mental health difficulty (van Wezel et al., 2023). This is made possible due to a process known as co-production – where both learned and lived experience knowledge fuses together to form a more complete interpretation of a situation and/or phenomena (for more information, see Section 5.4) (Brown et al., 2020).

For a more hands-on approach to influencing service delivery, Irish services also encourage user involvement through the creation of local forums. These are groups comprised of those who use services, their family members/carers/supporters and service providers. These groups were set up to support service improvement through dialogue between all stakeholders. Finally, user involvement can also occur at the research phase of service development through the inclusion of Patient and Public Involvement [PPI] representatives. PPI is beneficial in research as it ensures that the research that is carried out will make a unique, meaningful and cost-effective contribution to the end user (Arumugam et al., 2023). In relation to insight, through the service user's access to all the above resources, they are able to utilise their knowledge, based on lived experience to benefit their own care, the care of others and indeed benefit to the service itself. Such benefits to the organisation will now be presented.

5.3.2. Benefits of User Involvement to the Organisation

User involvement also has a number of benefits to the organisation that embeds such practices. Firstly, in recent years, policy, frameworks and legislation have advocated for service users to be involved in service provision. In allowing user involvement to occur, the organisation is adhering to and compliant with the quality standards that are laid out within such documentation (Batalden et al., 2016). In terms of patient flow, allowing service users to be involved in service provision beyond the patient identity helps reduce the rates of emergency department admissions and psychiatric ward admissions by between 30% and 50% (Spencer et al., 2013). As such, service user involvement is noted to improve service delivery which inherently improves service outcomes (OECD, 2011). A rationale for this may be that the service user gets a sense of ownership of both the service and their own recovery (Pestoff, 2013). As a result of this, user involvement can be seen as the bridge between the standards required by research and the realities of practice (Starkey & Maden, 2001). However, there is still a lack of evidence to identify if these benefits transcend into long-term benefits or not and thus this warrants further empirical investigation (Ezaydi et al., 2023).

5.4. Co-production

Co-production is a term that can be conceptualised in many different ways and as such has no universal definition (Masterson et al., 2022). However, for the purposes of this text, the definition we will abide by comes from the work of Norton (2022). According to Norton (2022) co-production is defined as:

> the creation and continuous development of a dialogical space
> where all stakeholders, including service users, family members,

carers, supporters and service providers enter a collaborative partnership with the aim of not only improving their own care but also that of service provision. (p. 27)

In this sense, co-production involves equality within this collaborative relationship, to the extent that if this was not in place, the co-productive activity would fail. Despite co-production not having a universal definition, the process is said to involve co-design, co-governance, co-implementation and co-evaluation (Health Service Executive, 2018). In this way, co-production captures the whole engagement process from its design right way through to its eventual evaluation.

Co-production originated at the University of Indiana in the 1970s within the field of economics when Elinor Ostrom and her team tried to decipher why crime increased when policemen on the streets were replaced with police vehicles (Norton, 2019, 2022). Since then, it has grown significantly across disciplines, invading spaces within economics, law, public management and now health care. Within this space, co-production has a number of principles. These were first coined by Edgar Cahn when he used co-production within the legal system to create think tanks. Here, Cahn (2000) identified the four fundamental principles of co-production as:

1. Recognising people as assets,
2. Valuing work differently,
3. Promoting reciprocity,
4. Building social capital.

The principles of co-production have increased substantially since Cahn's first interpretation of them (Norton, 2022). However, these four principles have lasted the test of time and are still fundamental in the practice of co-production today.

Today, within an Irish context, mental health policy and frameworks now promote user involvement and co-production. For instance, within the national policy document: '*Sharing the Vision*', user involvement is promoted by the creation of working groups, made up of all stakeholders, to implement the various recommendations stated in the policy (Department of Health, 2020). Additionally, this ethos of user involvement has transcended down to service frameworks and guidelines like: '*A National Framework for Recovery in Mental Health*' and its next iteration '*A National Framework for Mental Health Recovery*' where user involvement and co-production are imperative to the achievement of the ideals documented by these frameworks (Health Service Executive, 2017, *In Press*).

5.5. Conclusion

In summary, this chapter examined the concepts of user involvement and co-production. Models of user involvement are explored through the Arnsteins ladder of participation and MHERs engagement continuum. The importance of user involvement for both the individual and the organisation is then discussed followed by the concept of co-production in detail. Co-production principles are explored, stating their origins with Edgar Cahn to the numerous principles there are today. Finally, co-production and user involvement placement within a policy context is examined, particularly as it relates to both '*Sharing the Vision*' and '*A National Framework for Recovery in Mental Health*'. The next chapter of this text will move away from user involvement to examine the relationship between society since the foundation of the state to that of mental health, addiction and dual diagnosis.

References

Aase, I., Ree, E., Johannessen, T., Holen-Rabbervik, E., Thomsen, L. H., Stromme, T., Ullebust, B., Schibevaag, L., Lyng, H. B., O'Hara, J., & Wiig, S. (2021). Strategies and lessons learnt from user involvement in researching quality and safety in nursing homes and homecare. *International Journal of Health Governance*, *26*(4), 384–396. https://doi.org/10.1108/IJHG-05-2021-0044

Arumugam, A., Philips, L. R., Moore, A., Kumaran, S. D., Sampath, K. K., Migliorini, F., Maffulli, N., Ranganadhababu, B. N., Hegazy, F., & Botto-van Bemdem, A. (2023). Patient and public involvement in research: A review of practical resources for young investigators. *BMC Rheumatology*, *7*(1), 2. https://doi.org/10.1186/s41927-023-00327-w

Arnstein, S. (1969). A ladder of citizen participation. *Journal of the American Institute of Planners*, *35*(4), 216–224. http://dx.doi.org/10.1080/01944366908977225

Batalden, M., Batalden, P., Margolis, P., Seid, M., Armstrong, G., Opipari-Arrigan, L., & Hartung, H. (2016). Co-production of healthcare services. *BMJ Quality and Safety*, *25*(7), 509–517. https://doi.org/10.1136/bmjqs-2015-004315

Brown, M., & Jones, N. (2021). Service user participation within the mental health system: Deepening engagement. *Psychiatric Services*, *72*(8), 963–965. https://doi.org/10.1176/appi.ps.202000494

Brown, M., Pahl, K., Rasool, Z., & Ward, P. (2020). Co-producing research with communities: Emotions in community research. *Global Discourse*, *10*(1), 93–114. https://doi.org/10.1332/204378919X15762351383111

Cahn, E. (2000). *No more throw away people: The co-production imperative*. Essential Books.

Connaught Telegraph. (2020). *Bealach nua – supporting families of people with mental health difficulties*. https://www.con-telegraph.ie/2020/12/08/bealach-nua-supporting-families-of-people-with-mental-health-difficulties/

Cooper, Z., Cleary, S., Stelmach, W., & Zheng, Z. (2023). Patient engagement in perioperative settings: A mixed method systematic review. *Journal of Clinical Nursing*, *32*(17–18), 5865–5885. https://doi.org/10.1111/jocn.16709

Department of Health. (2020). *Sharing the vision: A mental health policy for everyone*. https://assets.gov.ie/76770/b142b216-f2ca-48e6-a551-79c208f1a247.pdf

Ezaydi, N., Sheldon, E., Kenny, A., Buck, E. T., & Weich, S. (2023). Service user involvement in mental health service commissioning, development and delivery: A systematic review of service level outcomes. *Health Expectations*, *26*(4), 1453–1466. https://doi.org/10.1111/hex.13788

Health Service Executive. (2017). *A national framework for recovery in mental health 2018–2020*. https://www.hse.ie/eng/services/list/4/mental-health-services/mental-health-engagement-and-recovery/resources-information-and-publications/national-framework-for-recovery-in-mental-health.pdf

Health Service Executive. (2018). *Co-Production in practice guidance document 2018–2020*. https://www.hse.ie/eng/services/list/4/mental-health-services/advancingrecoveryireland/

national-framework-for-recovery-in-mental-health/co-production-in-practice-guidance-document-2018-to-2020.pdf

Health Service Executive. (2023a). *Strategic plan 2023–2026: Engaged in recovery.* https://www.hse.ie/eng/services/list/4/mental-health-services/mental-health-engagement-and-recovery/mher-strategic-plan-engaged-in-recovery.pdf

Health Service Executive. (2023b). *Peer and family support.* https://www.hse.ie/eng/services/list/4/mental-health-services/mental-health-engagement-and-recovery/peer-and-family-support/

Health Service Executive. (2023c). *Better together: Health services patient engagement roadmap.* https://www.hse.ie/eng/about/who/national-services/partnering-with-patients/resourcesqid/hse-better-together-patient-engagement-roadmap-book.pdf

Health Service Executive. (In Press). A *national framework for mental health recovery.*

Hunt, E., & Byrne, M. (2019). *Peer support workers in mental health: A report on the impact of peer support workers in mental health services.* https://www.hse.ie/eng/services/list/4/mental-health-services/mental-health-engagement-and-recovery/peer-support-workers-in-mental-health-services.pdf

Kujala, S. (2008). Effective user involvement in production development by improving the analysis of user needs. *Behaviour and Information Technology, 27*(6), 457–473. https://doi.org/10.1080/01449290601111051

Lawn, S. (2015). Integrating service user participation in mental health care: What will it take? *International Journal of Integrated Care, 15*(4). https://doi.org/10.5334/ijic.1992

Masterson, D., Josefsson, K. A., Robert, G., Nylander, E., & Kjellstrom, S. (2022). Mapping definitions of co-production and co-design in health and social care: A systematic scoping review providing lessons for the future. *Health Expectations, 25*(3), 902–913 https://doi.org/10.1111/hex.13470

Naughton, L., Collins, P., & Ryan, M. (2015). *Peer support workers – A guidance paper.* https://www.lenus.ie/bitstream/handle/10147/576059/PeerSupportWorkersAGuidancePaper.pdf?sequence=6&isAllowed=y

Norton, M. (2019). Implementing co-production in traditional statutory mental health services. *Mental Health Practice, 27*(1). https://doi.org/10.7748/mhp.2019.e1304

Norton, M. (2022). *Co-production in mental health: Implementing policy into practice.* Routledge.

Norton, M. J. (2021). Co-production within child and adolescent mental health: A systematic review. *International Journal of Environmental Research and Public Health, 18*(22), 11897. https://doi.org/10.3390/ ijerph182211897

Norton, M. J. (2023). Peer support working: A question of ontology and epistemology. *International Journal of Mental Health Systems, 17*(1). 1. https://doi.org/10.1186/s13033-023-00570-1

OECD. (2011). *Together for better public services: Partnering with citizens and civil Society.* https://read.oecd-ilibrary.org/governance/together-for-better-public-services-partnering-with-citizens-and-civil-society_9789264118843-en#page1

Omeni, E., Barnes, M., MacDonald, D., Crawford, M., & Rose, D. (2014). Service user involvement: Impact and participation: A survey of service users and staff perspectives. *BMC Health Services Research, 14*, 491. https://doi.org/10.1186/s12913-014-0491-7

Pestoff, V. (2013). Collective action and the sustainability of co-production. *Public Management Review, 16*(3), 383–401. https://doi.org/10.1080/14719037.2013.841460

Starkey, K., & Maden, P. (2001). Bridging the relevance gap: Aligning stakeholders in the future of management research. *British Journal of Management, 12*(S1), S3–S26. https://doi.org/10.1111/1467-8551.12.s1.2

Spencer, M., Dineen, R., & Philips, A. (2013). *Co-producing services – co-creating health.* https://pdf4pro.com/amp/view/co-producing-services-co-creating-health-30be8.html

Tait, L., & Lester, H. (2005). Encouraging user involvement in mental health services. *Advances in Psychiatric Treatment, 11*(3), 168–175. https://doi.org/10.1192/apt.11.3.168

Tierney, E., McEvoy, R., O'Reilly-de Brun, M., de Brun, T., Okonkwo, E., Rooney, M., Dowrick, C., Rogers, A., & MacFarlane, A. (2014). A critical analysis of the implementation of service user involvement in primary care research and health service development using normalisation process theory. *Health Expectations, 19*(3), 501–515. https://doi.org/10.1111/hex.12237

van Wezel, M. M. C., Muusse, C., van de Mheen, D., Wijnen, B., den Hollander, W., & Kroon, H. (2023). What do we not know (yet) about recovery colleges? A study protocol on their (cost-) effectiveness, mechanism of action, fidelity and positioning. *BMC Psychiatry, 23*(1), 816. https://doi.org/10.1186/s12888-023-05293-8

Chapter 6

The Challenges of Mental Health, Addiction and Dual Diagnosis in an Irish Context

Oliver John Cullen[a] and Michael John Norton[b]

[a]*HSE Mental Health Services, Ireland*
[b]*HSE Office of Mental Health Engagement and Recovery, Ireland*

Abstract

Chapter 6 explores the cultural impact of mental health, addiction, and dual diagnosis challenges with a specific focus on Irish society. The chapter takes a staggered approach whereby each type of challenge is separated and discussed individually, before being joined together through discussions on dual diagnosis as presented in Section 6.4. These discussions are designed to highlight the cultural deviance that is perceived by other people towards those with such diagnosis over the years that such diagnosis have been prevalent in history. In particular, the discussions around dual diagnosis here will strengthen the discussion in Chapter 4: 'The Conundrum of Dual Diagnosis' and will set the groundwork for the remainder of this text.

Keywords: Culture; mental health; addiction; dual diagnosis; society

6.1. Introduction

Attitudes towards those with a mental health and/or an addiction challenge has shifted to various degrees in the past decade or so, with more people now utilising psychological support for their well-being than ever before (Blumner & Marcus, 2009; Mind, 2014). In this chapter, an exploration of the impact of mental health, addiction and dual diagnosis on Irish society will occur. This will allow

Different Diagnoses, Similar Experiences:
Narratives of Mental Health, Addiction Recovery and Dual Diagnosis, 57–62
Copyright © 2024 by Oliver John Cullen and Michael John Norton
Published under exclusive licence by Emerald Publishing Limited
doi:10.1108/978-1-80455-848-520241006

discussions on each of these challenges while also examining the nuances that make each of these challenges unique within service provision. Focus will also be given to the cultural impact on the individual, their family and the wider community. Dual diagnosis will also be briefly explored in order to strengthen understanding achieved in previous chapters as it relates to dual diagnosis. Section 6.2 commences this discussion by examining the cultural impact on mental ill health. This is followed by Section 6.3 which will explore the same, but in relation to addiction challenges. Section 6.4 explores the cultural impact of dual diagnosis followed by concluding remarks for this chapter in Section 6.5. Section 6.2 is now presented below.

6.2. Impact of Mental Ill Health

Our understanding of mental health has exploded in Irish society in recent years. What was once associated with '*danger*', '*fear*', '*lunatic*' and '*insane*' are now replaced by more positive associations including words like '*lived experience*', '*co-production*' and '*strength-based approach*' which are now used more regularly by both the services and the peers that were traditionally impacted by such stigmatising language. Such stigmatising language, in times gone by, was placed upon our neighbours, friends and relatives that were someway deviant from the norms of that time. However, thankfully, today we view these same individuals differently. Today, best practice stipulates that service users are now partners in the care process. This is achieved by the individual's taking personal responsibility for their own care plan (Mental Health Commission, 2012; Health Service Executive, 2021).

According to research carried out by academics at Maynooth University, National College of Ireland and Trinity College Dublin, 42% of Irish people at the time of the survey had a mental health disorder with more than 1 in 10 having attempted suicide (Maynooth University, 2022). With such stark figures, one can surmise that all families in Ireland are somehow impacted by mental health challenges. As such, not only is the individual affected by mental health challenges, but also the wider family. So how was this traditionally dealt with?

Since the Irish Republic was formed in 1922, Eamonn De Valera as Taoiseach and later, President of Ireland embraced a traditional Catholic approach to the family and what was deemed normal and abnormal in society. Anyone who fell outside of these set norms was normally institutionalised either in Mother and Baby Homes, traditional workhouses or mental asylums depending on the nature of the deviant act or behaviour (Dukelow & Considine, 2009; Norton, 2022). As for the mental asylums, history tells a very bleak tale of this time. Whilst institutions arose out of developments made in the 1800s, the establishment of these institutions continued well into the 20th century, supported by De Valera's ethos. From the 1950s onwards, advancements in the area of psychopharmacology and biomedicine saw mental distress being treated in a more humane fashion than what preceded this time. However, whilst the service had moved to a more therapeutic and humane interpretation of mental distress, society at large still held a stigmatising attitude towards such individuals.

More recently, a different interpretation of what constitutes mental distress and recovery came into being through the work of William Anthony (1993). Here he describes mental health recovery as '*a deeply personal, unique process of changing one's attitudes, values, feelings, goals, skills, and/or roles. It is a way of living a satisfying, hopeful and contributing life, even within the limitations caused by illness*' (p. 21). This work was later supported by Patricia Deegan who suggested that '*The goal of recovery is not to become normal. The goal is to embrace the human vocation of becoming more deeply, more fully human*' (Deegan, 1996, p. 92). Such new cultural understandings of mental distress and subsequent recovery suggests that one can live a full life even with the limitations of mental health challenges. Moreso than this, the lived experiences of mental distress that these individuals obtain are now seen as a type of knowledge that is readily sought in the treatment of mental health challenges (Norton, 2023). This change in perception of the mentally ill is slowly transcending to the remainder of society as more individuals are more willing to utilise mental health services today than they were decades earlier (Blumner & Marcus, 2009).

6.3. Impact of Addiction

Addiction is a contentious issue. From the side effects of excess alcohol use to the mind-altering impact of illegal drugs, mankind has always found a method for inebriation. Addiction does not discriminate between classes, colour or creed. It can happen to anyone at any stage of life. One drug most prominent in the Irish context is that of alcohol. In fact, temperance leader and priest Fr. Theobald Mathew, played a pivotal role in encouraging sobriety from the substance during his tenure in the 1800s. Throughout Ireland, his influence guided many to a life of temperance culminating in 1841, when his words and guidance supported a staggering 4.6 million people into sobriety (Britanica, 2023). Still somewhat influenced by Catholicism today, children from 11 to 12 years of age can take a pledge to not drink alcohol until they are 18. In the 1830s, the socio-economic, political and religious outlets all voiced concerns about the consumption of alcohol, describing it as '*socially deleterious*' – associating it with poverty and anti-social behaviours (Kelly, 2015). This issue became contentious during this time in Irish history, with negative assumptions towards the issue being taken by the leaders of the time. This time of debate did not last as during the 1960s, legislating the sale, supply and consumption of alcohol softened somewhat (Smyth et al., 2011).

We can't distinguish the cultural perception of Irish people as heavy drinkers from this discussion because it is observed as the norm in many parts of our culture. '*Uisce Beatha*' a term associated with whiskey, translates into '*Blessed water*'. The consumption of this whiskey has been a right of passage within Irish culture for centuries. With the decline of Catholic ideals in Ireland, so too has the notion of temperance from alcohol consumption. The 'pub' was now an Irish staple, ingrained into Irish society, used specifically for celebratory events and also for sad occasions, like funerals.

During the 1980s illegal drug use soared in Ireland, and with it, met societal distain. Drugs like heroin were now readily available within Irish society, and so too were diseases associated with their use. For example, HIV/AIDS. Despite the presence of these drugs, the lay population still could not correlate a causal relationship between Alcohol and street drugs. As a result, individuals with opiate addiction were often stigmatised more than those with alcohol addictions, called '*junkies*' and '*scumbags*', to the extent that some individuals would even self-identify as the same. In 2000, the Drug Misuse Research Division and the Health Research Board conducted a survey. One finding suggests that alcohol was more damaging than other, illegal, illicit substances. Interestingly, despite this conclusion, the majority of individuals would be uncomfortable in the company of a drug addict and a staggering 90% of 1,000 surveyed identified illegal drugs are a major issue within Irish society (Bryan et al., 2000).

In 2015, an amendment to the Misuse of Drugs Bill allowed for the legislation of supervised injection sites for intravenous drug users, with the purpose of harm reduction (National Social Inclusion Office, 2023). Planning permission has been granted for a facility in Dublin City but objections and concerns have caused delays. To date, this has not been put in place. In essence, Irish culture is far more tolerant than historically viewed. However, stigma within substances use still exist. An alcoholic drink in an expensive bar in an Irish city is a far cry from a back alley intravenous drug user, however they both may be trying to achieve the same outcome.

6.4. Impact of Dual Diagnosis

As previously mentioned, despite the fluidity in understanding what dual diagnosis is, for the purpose of this text, the term is simply defined as two co-occurring disorders – mental health and addiction challenges (Cullen & Norton, 2021). As described earlier in this chapter, we see examples of common issues that arise in both mental health and addiction, stigma being the most prevalent of both. So, if we look at the dynamic of both challenges running synchronously, such synchronicity can create more difficult and compounding issues for the individual impacted by dual diagnosis. The cyclic nature of addiction makes it difficult to treat, and mental health by its very nature is equally as complex and distressing. According to Farren et al. (2014), these co-occurring disorders are described as '*mutually detrimental*'. Through their study of 205 patients who had completed a dual diagnosis programme, the results over a 5-year time period concluded that psychopathology relating to depression, anxiety and cravings subsided (Farren et al., 2014). As a result, the text concluded that the disorders that make up a dual diagnosis challenge can be successfully treated together to obtain prolonged and lasting recovery over time (Farren et al., 2014).

Weaver et al. (2003) found that those with an illicit substance or alcohol-related addiction, had a high probability of experiencing a co-occurring mental health challenge. Although this study is 20 years old it is seminal as it shows the need for service reformation when it comes to treating dual diagnosis. Recently, the Health Service Executive launched a model of care for dual diagnosis, that supports the vision portrayed in '*Reducing Harm, Supporting Recovery 2017–2025*', '*Sharing the Vision: A Mental Health Policy for Everyone*' and '*Model of Care for People with Mental Disorder and Co-existing Substance Use Disorder (Dual Diagnosis)'* (Department of Health, 2017, 2020; Health Service Executive, 2023). The integration of these documents will support the reduction in stigma that still exists within society and services today. Treatment of dual diagnosis within services has the potential to save lives and support individuals and families to live a productive and harm-free life. However, more work is needed for this cultural change to become a reality.

6.5. Conclusion

This chapter can be summarised as a need to understand the complexities of mental health, addiction, and dual diagnosis from a cultural perspective. When society takes a stance of segregation and isolation, the individual who seeks recovery is often left outside the walls of societal norms. This creates an unhealthy bias towards the individual often demonstrated through the guise of stigma. Through knowledge and past experiences, the response of embracing recovery and offering individuals a pathway of hope and a future without disparity between individuals is crucial for society and service provision. When a hand reaches out in the dark, someone's life may be saved. Such experiences are now demonstrated in the sections that follow which will introduce the personal narratives of individuals at various stages of recovery from mental health, addiction, and dual diagnosis challenges. These inspirational stories are now presented.

References

Anthony, W. A. (1993). Recovery from mental illness: The guiding vision of the mental health service system in the 1990s. *Psychosocial Rehabilitation Journal, 16*(4), 11–23. https://doi.org/10.1037/h0095655

Bryan, A., Moran, R., Farrell, E., & O'Brien, M. (2000). Drug-related knowledge, attitudes and beliefs in Ireland: Report of a nation-wide survey. *Drug Misuse Research Division, Health Research Board.* https://www.hrb.ie/fileadmin/publications_files/KABREPORT.pdf

Blumner, K. H., & Marcus, S. C. (2009). Changing perceptions of depression: Ten-year trends from the general social survey. *Psychiatric Services, 60*(3), 306–312. https://doi.org/10.1176/ps.2009.60.3.306

Britanica. (2023). *Theobald Matthew.* https://www.britannica.com/biography/Theobald-Mathew

Cullen, O. J., & Norton, M. J. (2021). Chicken or egg: A dual diagnosis narrative. *Journal of Psychiatric and Mental Health Nursing, 29*(4), 507–511. https://doi.org/10.1111/jpm.12801

Deegan, P. (1996). Recovery as a journey of the heart. *Psychiatric Rehabilitation Journal, 19*(3), 91–97. https://doi.org/10.1037/h0101301

Department of Health. (2017). *Reducing harm, supporting recovery: A health-led response to drug and alcohol use in Ireland 2017–2025.* http://www.drugs.ie/downloadDocs/2017/ReducingHarmSupportingRecovery2017_2025.pdf

Department of Health. (2020). *Sharing the vision: A mental health policy for everyone.* https://assets.gov.ie/76770/b142b216-f2ca-48e6-a551-79c208f1a247.pdf

Dukelow, F., & Considine, M. (2009). *Irish social policy: A critical introduction*. Policy Press.

Farren, C. K., Murphy, P., & McElroy, S. (2014). A 5-year follow-up of depressed and bipolar patients with alcohol use disorder in an Irish population. *Alcoholism: Clinical and Experimental Research, 38*(4), 1049–1058. https://doi.org/10.1111/acer.12330

Health Service Executive. (2021). *Writing a person-centred individual care plan guidance document*. https://www.hse.ie/eng/services/list/4/mental-health-services/individual-care-plans/hse-good-individual-care-plans.pdf

Health Service Executive. (2023). *Model of care for people with mental disorder and co-existing substance use disorder (dual diagnosis)*. https://www.hse.ie/eng/about/who/cspd/ncps/mental-health/dual-diagnosis-ncp/dual-diagnosis-model-of-care.pdf

Kelly, J. (2015). The consumption and sociable use of alcohol in eighteenth-century Ireland. *Proceedings of the Royal Irish Academy Section C Archaeology, Celtic Studies, History, Linguistics, Literature, 115C*, 219–255. https://doi.org/10.3318/PRIAC.2015.115.14

Maynooth University. (2022). *Over 40% of Irish adults have a mental health disorder and one in ten have attempted suicide – MU, NCI and Trinity College Research*. https://www.maynoothuniversity.ie/news-events/over-40-irish-adults-have-mental-health-disorder-and-one-ten-have-attempted-suicide-mu-nci-and

Mental Health Commission. (2012). *Mental health commission guidance document on individual care planning mental health services*. https://www.mhcirl.ie/sites/default/files/2021-01/Guidance%20Document%20on%20Individual%20Care%20Planning.pdf

Mind. (2014). *Survey shows greatest improvement in public attitudes to mental health in 20 years*. https://www.mind.org.uk/news-campaigns/news/survey-shows-greatest-improvement-in-public-attitudes-to-mental-health-in-20-years/

National Social Inclusion Office. (2023). *Supervised injecting facilities*. https://www.hse.ie/eng/about/who/primarycare/socialinclusion/addiction/supervised-injecting-centre/

Norton, M. (2022). *Co-production in mental health: Implementing policy into practice*. Routledge.

Norton, M. J. (2023). Peer support working: A question of ontology and epistemology? *International Journal of Mental Health Systems, 17*(1). https://doi.org/10.1186/s13033-023-00570-1

Smyth, B. P., Kelly, A., & Cox, G. (2011). Decline in age of drinking onset in Ireland, gender and per capita alcohol consumption. *Alcohol and Alcoholism, 46*(4), 478–484. https://doi.org/10.1093/alcalc/agr047

Weaver, T., Madden, P., Charles, V., Stimson, G., Renton, A., Tyrer, P., Barnes, T., Bench, C., Middleton, H., Wright, N., Paterson, S., Shanahan, W., Seivewright, N., Ford, C., & Comorbidity of Substance Misuse and Mental Illness Collaborative Study Team. (2003). Comorbidity of substance misuse and mental illness in community mental health and substance misuse services. *British Journal of Psychiatry, 183*, 304–313. https://doi.org/10.1192/bjp.183.4.304

Part 2

Mental Health

Chapter 7

Diagnosed Disconnect – Prescribed Harm

Michaela Mc Daid

Introduction

I love to write, having previously shared my lived experience of mental health in articles, essays and talks. I've always focused on emotional hurt and healing with only passing reference to diagnosis. I welcome the opportunity to contribute to this book as the theme allows me to examine the impact that diagnosis and subsequent treatment had on my recovery. As a personal narrative, what follows is not an argument for or against diagnoses or treatment choices for other people. I simply relay my own experience and interpretation of it, as only I am qualified to do.

The Beginning – A Very Good Place to Start

To highlight the most glaring omission of psychiatric diagnosis, I will briefly share my backstory as a starting point. Surely, this is important to understand any story. Traits of my character, relevant to '*mental health challenges*' were evident in early childhood. I was always highly intuitive, empathic and sensitive. As a perfectionist and high achiever, I was self-critical, readily accepting responsibility to make things better. I was also intelligent and creative. An active mind, unbound by the realms of possibility, meant my imagination provided escape from any hurt I felt. Possibly because of these traits, insomnia, vivid dreams and nightmares are some of my most abiding childhood memories.

My formative years were punctuated by changing environments, from conflict in Northern Ireland, to the outback of Australia, to boarding school and back to rural Ireland by age 14. Assimilation and making new friends were survival skills that I mastered with outgoing confidence and an affable personality. While my immediate family was fractured by alcohol and boarding school, emigration also meant absence of a wider family circle. I always had a sense of aloneness and fitting in rather than belonging.

Different Diagnoses, Similar Experiences:
Narratives of Mental Health, Addiction Recovery and Dual Diagnosis, 65–75
Copyright © 2024 by Michaela Mc Daid
Published under exclusive licence by Emerald Publishing Limited
doi:10.1108/978-1-80455-848-520241007

Many will recognise these as Adverse Childhood Experiences [ACE's], factors increasing the risk of mental illness. Despite this, or maybe because of it, I reflect on a child who was adept at coping with challenges and change. She was both sociable and comfortable in solitude. She felt deeply, expressed emotions freely, and knew instinctively to seek comfort in nature and imagination when necessary.

Just Add Trauma

I was becoming a teenager when I returned to Ireland with my parents and only sister. My two older brothers remained in Australia and London. Within two years of being home, my big sister, whom I adored, killed herself. She was 18, I was 16. I resuscitated her on the side of a road, but she still died. I was in shock and couldn't grieve. Instead, I did what I knew best, I moved again. By the end of that summer, I had relocated from rural Ireland to inner city London. I enrolled myself in secondary school and excelled academically and in sports. I disconnected from the tragedy by creating a brand-new life, forming new relationships with people who knew nothing of my past. I chose not to tell them.

Mix in Life Stressors and Respond Naturally

While studying for A Levels[1] and applying to universities, I became pregnant. I continued to study, while also working to support myself and my son as a 19-year-old single parent. Physically, I was extremely fit and healthy. Mentally, I was resilient and resourceful. Understandably, I still felt the strain of sleep deprivation, isolation and financial pressure. I was coping, but acknowledged that I was starting to struggle. So, wanting the best for my son, I did the responsible thing – I sought help. The messaging was clear, '*seeking help*' meant seeing a GP. So, that's what I did.

Voila! A Diagnosis

This is where my story will be frighteningly familiar to many. In London in 1995, a 7-minute consultation with an NHS[2] GP I was meeting for the first time, resulted in a diagnosis of depression and prescription for psychotropic medication. There was no context to why I was feeling the way I was, no mention of ACEs, trauma, grief, or stressful living conditions, no signposting practical support or talking therapy. A medical diagnosis with pharmaceutical treatment was my only option. That was that. I was 22.

---

[1]A Level (Advanced Level) is a subject-based qualification conferred as part of the General Certificate of Education offered by the educational bodies in the United Kingdom to students completing secondary or pre-university education, usually at age 17/18.
[2]National Health Service – The umbrella term for the publicly funded health system in the UK.

How Diagnosis Felt, What It Meant to Me

At this stage of my life, so much had happened so quickly that I was in a kind of survival mode just to get through each day. I had already escaped painful feelings by moving, overworking and overachieving. Now, I had a medical diagnosis and treatment reinforcing the notion that numbing emotional pain was the right thing to do. The diagnosis told me that feelings of sadness, anxiety and overwhelm weren't a natural response to difficult life events, because these events hadn't been mentioned. Instead, my emotional response was framed as malfunctioning. This was a physiological issue, a chemical imbalance in my brain that could only be rectified medically, with a chemical cure.

I was a fitness instructor who didn't drink alcohol, smoke cigarettes, or use any other substances because health was important to me. I understood that using substances to cope could lead to dependency and more issues. But when a medical professional acknowledged my suffering with criteria of symptoms and a diagnosis, being prescribed drugs felt like validation. I had barely taken paracetamol before this point, so taking drugs daily felt like a big step, and one that I'd rather not take. But I was assured that this was a short-term, necessary treatment for my illness. There was no information on side effects, potential harm, or dependency, and certainly no alternative offered. The point was to stop me from feeling, so I could keep going. So, that's what I did. I took the tablets, and I just kept going, and going and going.

Yet, no matter how hard I tried to avoid them, painful and necessary emotions kept coming up. When they did, I now understood them as *'symptoms of my illness'*. Therefore, not something to explore or share with family and friends. The only person qualified to treat the symptoms of an illness was a medical doctor. I still had a feeling that another way would be healthier, but without the financial means for private healthcare I couldn't explore other options. My sister had killed herself. I never wanted to get that hopeless, I had a young child depending on me. I had to do something. Without money, this was my only option, and at least it was something.

Uncomfortably Numb

You don't have to be medically trained to know that drugs can't selectively numb emotions. In numbing painful feelings, prescription drugs also anaesthetised all feelings. My intuition was blunted and my creative energy sapped. Anti-depressant medication was robbing me of these natural coping resources. I felt worse. Each visit to the psychiatrist resulted in medications being changed and/or increased. I began to think I'd never get better, and my latest diagnosis of a *'severe, recurring, treatment resistant, depressive disorder'* reinforced my resignation. The treatment for this new diagnosis was to keep increasing the dosage until I was utterly disconnected from myself, just as life kept piling on the stress.

During this time, I had moved back to Northern Ireland, moving house 5 times in as many years. I lost both parents suddenly, and a disproportionate number of friends and family died by suicide. I was in an abusive relationship and had the relentless financial pressure of single parenthood. But I just kept going, feeling very little – crying not at all.

Not so Pretty – Polypharmacy

Instead of being felt and expressed, profoundly important emotions were numbed and buried deeper, to fester into psychosomatic illness. My prescription widened to include medications for irritable bowel syndrome and migraine. So-called 'side effects' crept up gradually, weren't initially connected to the psychotropic medication in my system and became ever-present. I gained a huge amount of weight despite a healthy diet and fitness regime, this affected my self-esteem. I had a tremor, itchy skin and constant thirst, this affected my social skills. When I tried to discuss these issues with medical prescribers, they were dismissed as *'just side effects'* and I was offered *'something to help with that'*, meaning more drugs to stop my body from reacting to the drugs it was already struggling to process.

In reality, there's no such thing as *'side effects'*; there are just effects. Some are desirable – I didn't feel overwhelming sadness anymore. Some are undesirable – I had to avoid eating in company and ran to the toilet constantly. As a result, I became socially anxious, I withdrew, and my mental health worsened.

Hurray! Now I'm Bipolar

The more anti-depressants silenced my sadness and stifled my creativity, the more creatively these vital parts of me sought expression, through suicidal ideation and psychosis. I had always felt deeply, with visceral bodily responses to my emotions and environment, but accepted this was just how I experienced the world. But after taking heavy doses of anti-depressant medication for a long period of time, these experiences became extreme, forceful and frightening. Sadness became sinister and I experienced delusions and hallucinations. I was re-diagnosed with bipolar affective disorder and hospitalised – twice. Psychiatrists explained this as a severe, lifelong illness, probably hereditary. As such, I would have to accept the limitations it placed on my life. After many years of the drugs not working, this re-diagnosis brought a sense of relief. It explained what was really wrong with me. I wasn't 'depressed' all along, I was bipolar! So now, with the right diagnosis, I would finally get the right medication, so I could be well.

I was awarded Disability Living Allowance to reiterate that with this more serious diagnosis, employment was unrealistic. My prescription was now an anti-depressant, anti-anxiety, mood stabiliser, anti-psychotic and sleeping medication – daily. This was a maintenance dose. I wasn't 40 yet.

Be a Good Girl, Take Your Medicine

I remained compliant because I equated compliance with being responsible. These were medical experts, and I had a diagnosable illness. They must know better than my own sense that I'd prefer not to be on a cocktail of drugs for the rest of my life. But remember, I was poor, so didn't have the privilege of treatment choice and couldn't afford therapy. I became resigned to a half-life and for the first time started using alcohol and cannabis to sleep, socialise, feel and not feel. I was already disconnected, medicated and reduced to a passive existence, so why not?

At this time powerful, anti-stigma campaigns were increasing in the media. Questioning or resisting a bipolar diagnosis and lifetime of medication was portrayed as being unnecessarily embarrassed or ashamed of an illness. This illness was akin to any physical illness, not my fault and out of my control. Yet, I was still aware that I had never grieved the loss of those I loved most in the world, and my current circumstances were still undeniably tough. When I stripped it all back, the fact remained that I was medicating my emotions. As little as I felt, that still just didn't feel quite right.

Working to Educate Young Minds

Having excelled academically through it all, I couldn't accept a life not using my brain. So, starting in a voluntary capacity and progressing to a full-time coordinator role, I carved out a successful career in mental health education. I worked for charities delivering mental health awareness courses to a broad cross-section of society. These courses were devised in-house with clinical governance and approval of the board. The chair of the board was a psychiatrist. Most of my work was in schools.

I delivered PowerPoint presentations on mental health and illness, including a video, aimed at teenagers on how SSRI's[3] worked. The penultimate slide, taking 5 minutes of a 90-minute session, was dedicated to '*self-help*' and '*alternative*' or '*complementary*' therapies. Language is important and the message was loud and clear; the medical model is the credible main event, everything else is secondary. '*Reduce stigma!*' was the catchphrase. This effectively meant 'if you're struggling see your GP, get a diagnosis, and comply with medical treatment'.

Lived experience made my delivery very convincing. I was holding down a good job, despite serious mental illness. I spoke about how medication had saved me and was absolutely necessary for managing bipolar affective disorder. I was teaching young teenagers that feelings of depression and anxiety at this difficult stage of development weren't '*normal*' responses, but diagnosable medical illness, treated by doctors, with medication. I had become part of the problem.

Listening More Than Talking

As well as working with teenagers, I facilitated countless groups of adults from vastly different backgrounds. I used this position to listen as much as I talked, and learn as much as I taught by asking groups to consider for themselves '*What helped?*'. A very definite pattern emerged from responses; '*the garden. … my pet…*

---

[3]Selective serotonin reuptake inhibitors (SSRIs) are a widely used type of antidepressant.

fishing … .a good walk'. I was teaching the importance of seeking professional, medical help and diagnosis. Yet, without direction and irrespective of background, hundreds of people repeatedly told me that at times of distress, they were drawn to nature.

Hold on a Minute!

This was my '*Hold on a minute!* Moment'. I reflected on my own relationship with nature. As a child in the Australian outback, I instinctively '*went bush*', alone with my dog when I was upset. When struggling in London as a teenager and young adult, I took long walks on Hampstead Heath. Even as a suicidal inpatient of a Northern Ireland psychiatric hospital, I gazed out the window, yearning to be in the small wooded area beside the hospital. It was true! The more distressed I had felt, the stronger the pull to be with nature.

So, countless strangers were telling me nature helped them, my own experience told me that nature helped me. But I was personally and professionally enmeshed in a medical model of diagnosis and drugs, so I knew that the mental health system gave no credence to the importance of nature connection for good mental health. Why not?

Since that first GP appointment, I had been a model patient accepting every diagnosis and taking every medication prescribed, as prescribed. Despite long waiting lists, I always attended appointments and engaged fully. The fact that my prescription had only ever increased was surely a clear indication that it wasn't working. I had lost faith. I had to disengage from the mental health system, ironically, for the good of my mental health.

At this juncture, it's important to remind readers that I had spent 20 years in mental health education. I was well-informed and acutely aware of risks associated with what I was doing. As a patient with a diagnosis of bipolar and a history of psychosis and suicidal ideation, wanting to stop medication would be interpreted as '*lacking insight*' and '*non-compliance with treatment*'. Understandably, no psychiatrist would agree in case I killed myself on their watch. I had to do this myself, carefully and sensibly. I kept a diary of my mood and symptoms, telling one close friend who I saw regularly and trusted completely. She had a key to my house, details of my GP and psychiatrist, and my written consent to intervene if mood changes and/or behaviours became alarming or dangerous.

While very gradually tapering medication, I increased self-awareness and nature connection. I slowed down; making life choices that prioritised well-being above productivity and finances. I moved to the countryside and immersed myself in nature, turning the soil, walking the hills, and swimming in the cold sea. Long before sea swimming was popularised by lockdown and the scientific evidence of mental health benefits became common knowledge, I was drawn to the cold because it felt like a reset. In withdrawal from drugs, cold water was clean, fresh and pure. I was outdoors, usually barefoot, in all weather.

I didn't know then that this was *Ecotherapy*, and I was in intensive care. I hadn't done any research and had no professional input. I was guided entirely by my intuition and felt sense of what soothed and what agitated me, choosing behaviours and environments accordingly. Through nature, I reconnected with the raw, hurting version of myself that never had a voice. In solitude, I sobbed and wailed from the depth of my being, held with acceptance, love and support by other-than-human nature. I also experienced surges of ecstasy and high energy, which I allowed to flow through me without fear. I felt, processed and released a lifetime of grief and emotional pain, and I healed.

What Would the Doctor Say?

Can you imagine if I had told my psychiatrist that I was getting into the cold sea in winter and had stopped wearing shoes? I touched and talked to trees, listening to what they had to tell me. I wrote frenzied non-sensical streams of consciousness in the middle of the night. I danced freely whenever I felt the urge to move and shake my body. Without understanding why, I tapped my fingertips on my head and face to relieve tension. I tuned into the cycles of the moon and seasons and followed their rhythm. Although these behaviours are strange in the 21st century mainstream Western world, they made me feel better, lighter, more balanced and grounded. I had a sense of reconnection to myself as part of the natural world. I became more confident and capable in all aspects of my life. Yet, had I tried to explain this to a psychiatrist in a typical 10-minute consultation, s/he would have taken one look at my bulging file and concluded that I was hypo-manic, elated, delusional, hallucinating, psychotic. These healing and nourishing, though unconventional behaviours would have been classed as symptoms of an illness and stopped, with medication.

Within 2 years I was entirely medication-free, with no depression, elation, anxiety or psychosis. I was sleeping soundly, flourishing creatively, and enjoying better mental and physical health than I had ever known or dared believe possible.

With newfound clarity and a sense of epiphany, I requested my medical records to study them alongside my diaries. I objectively examined the timeline of how a healthy, hardworking 22-year-old, who experienced trauma and difficult life circumstances, became a heavily medicated, hospitalised bipolar patient before the age of 40. The answer is the *'treatment'* I received through psychiatric diagnosis. The correlation was clear. As bad as I had felt, I never had suicidal thoughts or psychosis before I took anti-depressants. Once labelled in a system that reduces human experience and emotional suffering to a checklist of DSM[4] symptoms,

---

[4]The *Diagnostic and Statistical Manual of Mental Disorders* (DSM; latest edition: DSM-5-TR, published in March 2022) is a publication by the American Psychiatric Association (APA) for the classification of mental disorders using a common language and standard criteria.

I may have survived and functioned, but only as a dumbed-down and subdued version of myself. I never would have thrived, re-claiming my passion, creativity and voice, with courage to share it with the world.

It's an Ecotherapy Life for Me

I was motivated to return to work in mental health, but only in a role that supported a holistic approach that valued education, self-determination and connection. My experience had taught me the importance of authenticity. I need to believe 100% in what I'm doing, otherwise I can't do it, not for convenience, money or status. Being out of alignment with my true self literally makes me sick.

I now work part-time for Solas Donegal in the Republic of Ireland. Solas is a mental health recovery programme based on a model of walking, talking and listening in green spaces. As a HSE[5]/IDP[6] partnership, referrals come from GPs, psychiatrists and psychologists. My colleague is a mental health nurse, liaising effectively with these professionals regarding diagnosis and medication. Referrals also come from social prescribers and self-referrals. As a Peer Support Worker, I promote ecotherapy, education, and community involvement.

We're not based in a clinical setting, but in a community building, from where we are outdoors and active. Participants with a broad range of mental health challenges engage for 1, 2 or 3 days a week for 2 years. All aspects of the programme are co-produced by participants and staff. Each participant is valued as a unique individual with talents and skills, as well as psychiatric diagnoses and repeat prescriptions. We know each person's story because we listen and build a relationship. Solas participants are the agents of their own recovery, as staff we walk alongside them, providing support on their journey.

My role in Solas provides me with training in Ecotherapy and opportunities to network with other mental health professionals working outside the medical model. Instead of mental illness, diagnosis and medication, my understanding of mental health now focuses on being trauma informed and listening to emotional distress. This makes sense to me.

I am also self-employed in my own Ecotherapy Practice, where I'm not the therapist – nature is. I facilitate groups providing education and removing barriers to practical experiences in walking, hiking, sea swimming, forest bathing and bushcraft. I elevate the importance of nature for healing by creating time and space for this connection to be remembered and revalued. Then, I step back and

[5]Health Service Executive (HSE) (Irish: *Feidhmeannacht na Seirbhíse Sláinte*) is the publicly funded healthcare system in Ireland, responsible for the provision of health and personal social services. It came into operation on 1 January 2005.
[6]Inishowen Development Partnership (IDP) is a community led local development company delivering rural development and social inclusion programmes and initiatives in Donegal since 1996 on behalf of the European Union and the Irish Government through the National Development Plan.

let it happen naturally. My approach is intentionally and unapologetically simple. Layers of bureaucracy and professional hierarchy are stripped away to focus energy on innate human need: connection to nature, others and self. People crave time to slow down and space to be heard, so that's what I provide.

Personally, I continue to prioritise nature connection as a cornerstone of mental and physical health. My 'hold on a minute moment' was 9 years ago. Since then, my work in Ecotherapy has grown from strength to strength. I also write, study and travel. I swim in the sea and climb mountains. I enjoy healthy relationships with others and with myself. I'm 51 now and have never doubted for a second that heeding my intuition and disengaging from a medical model of mental health care was the best thing I could have done.

Ecotherapy is not some airy-fairy, hippy-dippy, new-age nonsense. It is a scientifically proven, evidence-based approach to mental health care that predates both psychotherapy and psychiatry. In recent years, Ecotherapy has gained recognition as a credible discipline due to an ever-increasing body of international research.[7] Science and academia are catching up with what intuition and lived experience always knew and told us, but we were too busy to listen – that nature heals.

Back to Basics – Not for Profit

Evolutionary psychology posits that all human emotions serve a purpose. Maybe, a reluctance to indefinitely aneaesthise emotions with drugs isn't a result of 'stigma'. Maybe, it's the result of something deeper, an innate knowing that feelings must be felt and expressed for human health. Intuition has been finely tuned over many millennia to keep us safe and well. It is not aligned with any interest other than ours.

My opinion is that the medicalisation of emotion can disempower individuals and disconnect communities. When emotional suffering is framed as an illness, it requires medical treatment by a qualified professional to '*make better*'. So, a person loses agency over their own wellbeing. The listening ear of friends, family and neighbours is devalued in the pursuit of symptoms, diagnosis, risk assessment and record-keeping. These are major concerns for the pressured professional, carrying a huge weight of responsibility. The result is that a vulnerable person, needing to be heard, talks to the top of a stranger's bowed head, because they're busy taking notes. The humanity of this human interaction is lost for both people.

It is transformational for a person to be fully present, listening to another person; not to intervene or fix, but to hold space for their pain with empathy and compassion. Yet the dominance of the medical model has deskilled and discouraged people from doing this for each other. They feel ill-equipped because they're not qualified professionals. With love and best intentions, family and friends are

---

[7]Construction and Initial Validation of the Reese EcoWellness Inventory (*International Journal for the Advancement of Counselling*, Vol. 37, No. 2, 2015).

now more inclined to respond to a person in distress by encouraging them to 'see someone about that', i.e. get on a waiting list for diagnosis and treatment. The professionalisation of support also means the natural feel-good factor of having helped someone in need, just by listening to them is denied to the layperson.

Despite media camapigns telling the public to 'seek professional help' for emotional suffering, there is still a reluctance to do so because people fear 'just being put on tablets'. This fear is not unfounded. It's the result of decades of disproportionate resources being invested in a medical model of mental health care.

Professionally and personally, I observe most people experiencing mental health challenges as a response to trauma, grief, abuse, inequality, discrimination, poverty, stress and isolation. So surely a connective human response, feeling heard and part of a just society with practical support would ease their distress. Instead, people are often 'on medication' indefinitely, as their only option, enabling them to tolerate the intolerable.

To each their own, respectfully

Polarisation of thought and opinion in any discourse is frustrating. I'm aware that my narrative may be manipulated and misrepresented as anti-medication and/or anti-psychiatry. The term 'pill shaming' is used to describe any viewpoint that questions the overuse of psychiatric medication and irresponsible prescribing practices. This is inaccurate and unhelpful. 'For or against' arguments disallow space for those in the middle, who are listening and weighing things up, with open, critical minds. Frankly, it's just not in my nature to shame anyone, least of all a person who is struggling and seeking support.

I fully understand and accept that for some, medication has been a useful short-term intervention to relieve the debilitating impact of mental health challenges. It has enabled lifestyle changes and engagement with support and talking therapies to address underlying issues. In turn, this has led to improved quality of life. Great! Equally, I accept and respect that for some, the long-term use of psychiatric medication is a well-informed choice, underlined by their lived experience. Also, great!

I do not judge or criticise the person seeking help, or the professional trying to provide that help. On this journey through diagnosis and treatment, I encountered well meaning, capable, ethical, overworked professionals. They did their best and did not mean to harm me. But they were doing their best in a broken system. Once diagnosed and medicated, my appointments were short, infrequent and seldom with the same person. Twice in 20 years, I was offered talking therapy; first, 6 × 1-hour sessions with a counsellor. Then, when I researched CBT[8] myself and requested it, I was on another waiting list for 18 months – taking medication all the while. I finally received an appointment, just as I was re-diagnosed with bipolar. A locum psychiatrist decreed that CBT was unsuitable for a bipolar patient.

---

[8]Cognitive Behavioural Therapy; a talking therapy focusing on managing problems by changing thoughts and behaviour.

My long-awaited therapy was cancelled with the stroke of a pen, and another prescription was written instead.

Conclusion

I conclude that diagnosis of mental illness, resulting in continuous treatment with copious amounts of psychotropic drugs was harmful to my mental and physical health. Painful, necessary emotions were numbed, so couldn't be processed and healed. I was disconnected from intuitive knowing that what I needed was time and safety to feel and express emotional pain. I found what I needed in the natural world.

The further I have distanced myself from a medical model of mental health care, the better my health has been. I've not only accepted, but grown to love my authentic self; that free-spirited, emotional, empathic, intuitive and nature-loving person I always was. I couldn't love myself while heavily medicated because I couldn't know myself.

As a personal essay, the relationship between government, psychiatry and the pharmaceutical industry is beyond the scope of this work. Suffice to say, I am convinced that this relationship had a direct bearing on how readily I was diagnosed with a '*severe lifelong psychiatric illness*', treatable with a lifetime's worth of pharmaceutical products. Without money, I was powerless to challenge this in a system built on power imbalance and profit, a system that has nothing to do with health and wellbeing.

I hope my story is heard amidst the multi-billion-pound campaigns to 'reduce the stigma of mental illness' by seeking and accepting diagnosis and medication in response to emotional pain. It is equally important that my story is heard alongside that of a person for whom diagnosis and medication was a positive experience. Everyone's experience is equally valid, but some are given more attention and credibility.

What if struggling 22-year-old me had the financial means to seek private healthcare? Drugs would never have been my first choice. Even without knowing what I do now, I would have chosen social and green prescribing and practical support. I would have engaged fully with counselling and psychotherapy. Then, I would never have known how bad things could get, and never had reason to share my story with you.

Chapter 8

A Well-Trodden Path

L. McGowan

Introduction

For this chapter, the term sexual violence is used as a blanket term that includes sexual assault of any kind, to anyone. According to the 2002 Sexual Abuse and Violence in Ireland (SAVI) report (McGee, 2002), 28% of the men and 42% of the women surveyed have experienced sexual violence at some point in their lives. Two Irish institutions conducted a study in 2018 to ascertain the current number of sexual violence victims in Ireland. Their research suggests that the prevalence of sexual violence was significantly higher than what the SAVI research had claimed. According to this survey, 15% of Irish adults have been raped (one in five women and one in ten men), and one in three adults have experienced some form of sexual violence (Vallières et al., 2020). In 2017, 2,945 victims bravely reported being a victim of sexual violence in Ireland (Recorded Crime Q4 2017, 2018). I was one of the 2,945. The account that follows sheds light on my ongoing journey toward recovery.

Alone

I don't know if my story will impact anyone, but I feel it needs to be told, even if just briefly. I wish I had known someone I could relate to or connect with through lived experience, to tell me what to expect, what to do, and what not to do, but maybe I wouldn't have listened anyway. On reflection, if I was to pick one feeling that was a common theme from the day it happened and even sometimes now, I would say loneliness.

My story to many will sound familiar. A story about a woman who was sexually assaulted by some guy: it's sad and shocking but for the most part, a few minutes after hearing about it, life moves on and we barely give it a second thought. That changes once that person is you. You are in a state of hypervigilance, you become extremely sensitive to your environment and every mention of anything related to sexual violence rings loud. And you remember, obsess, and

Different Diagnoses, Similar Experiences:
Narratives of Mental Health, Addiction Recovery and Dual Diagnosis, 77–84
Copyright © 2024 by L. McGowan
Published under exclusive licence by Emerald Publishing Limited
doi:10.1108/978-1-80455-848-520241008

dwell on it. At least I did anyway. There are so many of us out there – victims. We are everywhere, wandering together down this well-trodden path, but all the while wandering alone.

My story starts in 2017. Well, the events that led to my need for recovery began there. After a night out with friends I woke, groggy and hungover. For a few seconds, all I could think about was my headache. But slowly a feeling of dread smothered me. Memories of the events of the night before came flooding back. I needed medical attention, I was torn, metaphorically and physically. I called a friend. I didn't use the word rape, I just said there was blood, pain, and shattered glass. She encouraged me to go to the garda station (Ireland's National Police Service), so I did. The gardaí drove me to the Sexual Assault Treatment Unit (SATU), two hours away. This would be my first of four times in this unit. The attending forensic physician was male. The rape kit was carried out by him, in the presence of a nurse, while a guard stood on the other side of a drawn paper-thin curtain, for the chain of custody purposes I was told. The physician took photos of my naked body, '*for evidence*'.

The gardaí drove me home again late that night. As I watched them drive away, I walked in through my front door with the smashed glass panel, into my empty home. I sat on my couch, in shock, and pain, but all I felt was alone. I cried in a way I had never cried before. I was already mourning the person I used to be. She was gone and I knew she wasn't coming back. I was now forced to sit in the company of a stranger – myself. I did not know who I was.

The Aftermath

'*It's open and shut*'. Rightly or wrongly, that was what a guard said to me. There was so much evidence this was definitely going to court. The next few weeks were a haze of weekly visits to the station, adding onto statements, and getting updates. They confiscated my phone. Anybody I had any contact with the night it happened had to be interviewed by the gardaí. They told me they would give me a few days to talk to those closest to me so it could '*come from me*'. This amounted to over 15 people, 15 conversations and 15 times telling the people who loved and cared for me what had happened. A hard reality to face, that many times. But this turned out to be the first step towards recovery, I just didn't know it. When I started having to tell my story, I talked. I talked and talked and there was something in sharing the story that truly helped me. It was heartbreaking to see the hurt and pain in those looking back at me, but I started to feel like I wanted to scream my story to the world.

I was a single parent too. Every day trying to hide puffy, exhausted, sad eyes and transform me back into '*mammy*'. I can't describe how draining it was to not feel like me but have to pretend to be me. I missed myself so much. But you eat the darkness and bury it deep for your child. You hide it as best as you can so that the evil doesn't touch them in any way. So, you break beneath the surface instead.

In the weeks that followed every time I stepped outside, everything seemed deafeningly loud, but equally, it also felt like all sounds were muffled. It terrified me. I thought I was losing my mind. I walked around my local town searching for the faces of him and his family. I knew them, to see anyway. I thought I looked like a victim. I was sure when people glanced at me in passing that they knew I was a victim of sexual violence. They didn't, of course, but my paranoid mind wouldn't accept that. That paranoia grew. And before long I became paranoid about my closest family and friends. Hypervigilance is a common symptom for someone who has experienced trauma. They constantly search their surroundings for dangers maintaining a strong and perhaps obsessional awareness of their environment. I started to obsess about my state of mind, seeing him, the case, the court, and everything else related to what had happened.

I began to believe that many of my family members were involved in some conspiracy against me – meeting with the gardaí and my doctor behind my back. I was advised to attend the Rape Crisis Centre,[1] so I did. But I was too paranoid to go to my local centre so instead, each week, I travelled two hours away for my meeting. But this did not help with my paranoia. Lack of adequate sleep didn't help either, sleeping tablets turned me into a zombie. I wasn't coping and my counsellor suggested I visit my general practitioner (GP), so I did. I don't remember much of that visit but words such as post-traumatic stress disorder (PTSD), anxiety, and hyperarousal were used. I left with a follow-up appointment and a prescription.

During my initial visit to the SATU, the doctor administered a Hepatitis B injection (the first of three), emergency contraception, and preventative medication against chlamydia. Soon after I was on sleeping tablets for insomnia and antibiotics for my wounds as they had become infected. And now a prescription for anxiety, paranoia, and low mood. More unwanted things going into my body. I hated him! But my GP said I should take them, so I did.

Silence!

I felt weak and embarrassed being on medication and was reluctant to tell many about it. But after some time, I felt somewhat more capable and less paranoid. I began to trust my family again. I would visit a cousin regularly and I would talk to death about everything that happened, in great detail, step by step, sometimes for hours at a time. And I did this weekly, and it helped, more than she knows. However, most of the people I had initially told never mentioned it again and I really struggled with this, and still do at times. I understand it was probably mostly due to their discomfort or not knowing what to say but this reluctance to talk to me about it made me feel alone. I needed to keep the conversation going to allow me to process what had happened.

A friend told me about a Level Five Healthcare Assistant course and suggested I do it, so I did. I decided to do it as a distraction. My memory of that time is foggy. The course started just four months after I was assaulted. The first 4–5 months went by slowly and I never felt present. It was difficult studying being on sleeping tablets. Some evenings were spent in the garda station for a few hours,

---

[1]Rape Crisis Centre National 24-Hour Helpline: 1800 77 8888; E: info@rcc.ie; Website: https://www.drcc.ie/

then crying myself to sleep at night and having to face going to classes the next day seemed impossible. But I did my best and put on a brave face pretending all was good. Toward the end of the course, the lecturer suggested I continue my studies, so I did. I began my undergrad in social care that same year. I struggled all through the first year and was being treated for anxiety, PTSD, insomnia and depression. Every second week I would take a day off college and travel the four-hour round trip to the rape crisis centre. The case being built by the guards was ongoing and contact with them was very frequent. I was still struggling as a parent. It was all so smothering. But I realised that studying and getting up and going somewhere was the distraction I needed. The course also made me realise that I was learning to become part of a world much bigger than my own, I was learning to care for and respond to others who had their own struggles and vulnerabilities in life. This was a turning point in my life. Feeling stronger, at the beginning of my second year, I took a break from counselling.

During my second year in college, two years and seven months after my assault, two gardaí called to my house and asked me to come to the station. Something was wrong. I sat in the chair in a room I now knew like the back of my hand, and they told me that the Director of Public Prosecutions had decided on my case, and it would not be heard in court. I felt so small, childlike and alone sitting in the room that day. It was now the end of the legal road. I appealed. I lost. It was over. He would continue to walk free. I was told to name him publicly would be an offence and leave me open to a potential defamation case. I was silenced.

I returned to counselling, but this time in my local rape crisis centre. I threw myself into my studies and I focused on my daughter and myself. I followed the advice of my GP and took my medications as prescribed. I followed guidance from lecturers and worked hard when I could. I accepted the help of those who offered it and reached out when I felt I should. I made myself busy, so remarkably busy. I sometimes worked 60-hour weeks while raising my daughter and studying full-time. My coping mechanism was filling my life with so much there was little room for facing reality. Avoidance, my counsellor told me. Slow down!

Turning Something Meaningless into Something Meaningful

During my final year of college, I conducted research into the area of sexual violence. In addition to this, I also completed a course in peer support. I felt stronger and more focused. My medication was helping with intrusive and racing thoughts and my sleep was more regulated. I was more capable of managing triggers too. Although delving into the research topic was hard at times, I felt empowered as I saw a window of opportunity to turn my experiences into something positive. I worked hard for years without knowing if things would improve. But for the first time, I felt very hopeful about the future. I felt able to help others. Through my degree and research, I secured a place in a postgraduate course where I could further explore the area of sexual violence and I will hopefully be able to make a positive impact in this world for other victims. Everything happens for a reason, doesn't it?

The Things No One Tells You

For months after the assault, I searched the internet for written pieces, lived experience narratives, from victims in Ireland who re-laid their experiences so that I could learn about what to expect or whether what I was experiencing was normal. I wanted someone from Ireland because I thought at least the legal route would be somewhat similar and culturally we might have common beliefs, history, and understanding of what being a victim of sexual violence means in Ireland. But unfortunately, I was unable to source any adequate reading material to assist me. I have made note of only some issues that caused incredible stress and trauma in addition to the actual assault, in a bid to highlight for others that it is not just the events of that night that caused trauma, it was many of the things that followed too.

1.   When I first visited the Garda Station, they accompanied me to my house to get some belongings before I was brought to the SATU. They followed me to my bedroom, where the assault happened – more strangers in my home. They looked around my room, in drawers. In comparison to what had happened to me, this probably doesn't sound like a big deal, but it was humiliating. The guards walked around my bedroom slowly, taking it all in. I was then instructed to hand over the keys to my house so that the crime scene team could investigate my home. Someone in my home and I would not even be there. I obliged obviously, but it was all too much to process.

2.   When I was in the SATU, the physician, nurse and both gardaí sat with me in a meeting room. In this same room was a corner designed and decorated for children. It was filled with colourful children's books and toys. I will never forget looking at them all wondering how many children have sat in this room and worse, why they were there. That sight still haunts me. The physician opened a large booklet, filled with questions. Age/sex/date of birth/address etc. Normal things to begin with but then the questions become more personal, and intimate too. How much do I drink on a daily and weekly basis? Have I ever taken drugs? What contraceptives I was and am on if any? My whole complete sexual history – the good, the bad, and the ugly. Countless questions and I failed to understand why. To answer these questions to an audience of four strangers was humiliating, and traumatising. But I quietly and shamefully obliged.

3.   That first visit to the SATU was one of four. There are repeat visits for follow-up vaccinations and receiving test results. The unit test for HIV, syphilis, chlamydia, gonorrhoea and hepatitis B and C. Those visits ran over the course of seven months.

4.   The day after I reported the assault, I was asked to attend the station again. This time the garda told me I was to hand over my phone as part of the investigation. Initially, I refused, in a panic. I had personal, intimate content on my phone. I had been dating someone and thought it was a huge invasion of our privacy. When I declined to hand it over the sergeant was brought in and I was informed that either I hand it over there and then or they would seek a

court order and force me to. My heart was racing, tears streaming down my cheeks, frantically thinking of someone to call to come to help me, save me. This did not feel right. But with no one in my corner, I was defeated. And confused. How could the victim now be forced into doing something they did not want to? Surely, this was not right? That night the gardaí dropped me at my house again, the house I had been raped in, with no phone – no way to contact anyone. Alone! The following day the gardaí informed me that everything on my phone would be downloaded and could be used against me by the defence. Any conversations, photos or videos could be presented in court. In addition, they wanted access to the phones of the people I had been out with that night and to download our interactions in preparing for the night out. How could I ask people to hand over their phones to the gardaí? Surely this isn't right? But I have good family and friends, all but one gave their phones to the gardaí. But it was a hard task to face them and ask that of them.

5. In the months that followed I was encouraged to give written permission to the gardaí so they could write to my GP and my counsellor at the rape crisis centre and request my medical records and notes. I was told not giving permission may go against me in court. So, I obliged. The day my GP received the letter she rang me. They were requesting, without my prior knowledge, my full medical records dating back to my first period, over 20 years ago. They also asked how old I was when I began on birth control, whether I ever had any sexually transmitted infections, abortions, or miscarriages, and what type of birth I had with my daughter. They also asked have I had ever been prescribed any medication for any mental health-related issues. They wanted all the notes my counsellor had written about our sessions together. All the information gathered, I was told, could be used against me in court by the defence.

6. You are also not allowed to visit a solicitor or seek any legal advice. This may be construed as coaching in a courtroom and will most definitely go against you in court. Currently, in Ireland, the accused is represented by an expert, and experienced legal representatives and the victim has no legal representation for the trial (Irish Legal News, 2021). For those two years and seven months, I heard about what happened in that court setting. Normally, the victim, somehow, is blamed for the assault, and barristers and solicitors engage with you and point the finger at you. And presumably, your experience of engaging in a legal case is little to none. But you are not allowed to get any support or advice. You are alone.

7. No one tells you how threatening hospital and GP appointments will feel after an experience like this. Or going through airport security. Or how a million other relatively normal situations will make you feel abnormal.

8. Body memories. Any type of pain or ache in the pelvic region can recreate the pain of the original trauma.

9. Sexual trauma can have a physical impact on a person's health. I developed various, albeit mild, issues after my experience and continue to live with those side effects now.

Conclusion

The series of events laid out in this chapter are done so to give a brief insight into just how traumatising the whole legal process is as well as the assault itself. Every single event that day, and the months following, left deep and damning scars. I have heard numerous conversations of people discussing/judging some news report where a victim retracts her statement and I ask everyone to consider if it is any wonder. Two years and seven months of giving everything the garda needed to build a case. Being made vulnerable, exposed, defenceless, and unsafe, all in the name of bringing him to court. Open and shut, remember? All the trauma, humiliation, loneliness, tears, sleepless nights, hours and hours of statements, counselling, and medication. And for what? Now I had no choice but to face my reality with no distractions of a potential court case. Someone raped me!

One of my ongoing struggles is accepting that he is a part of my life, a hugely negative part, forever. For the rest of my days, I will know that my life has been affected by someone's choice to hurt me. All my stress, worries, tears and fears since then are because of him and there is no consequence for him. I am continuing to work on this, but even the fact that I must work on that is infuriating. My recovery journey is helping me find peace with this but it is a work in progress. However, I know I am fortunate to have an extremely supportive network. They are my recovery. And I am certain that the following are just some of the reasons I am in a better place now.

- Safety: Re-establishing safety and knowing who '*my people*' were.
- Being aware of my limits, especially in the early days. It was important that I felt safe and comfortable in my surroundings and often that meant avoiding, or leaving events, gatherings, and functions early to make that happen.
- Talking: It is not the trauma that makes us suffer emotionally but our inability to talk about it (Miller, 1981). Talking about what happened be it in talk therapy or with my partner, family members or friends helped me immensely. It needed to be someone I trusted. I did get that wrong once or twice but thankfully with no major consequences. Exploring what happened to me through talking with others helped me identify thoughts and behaviours I wanted and needed to change. Talking helped me face what happened to me, begin to learn to accept it, and work through it rather than allowing it to cause self-destruction.
- Helping others: Working with vulnerable people and being able to offer something positive back through volunteer work and my employment as a social care worker has been imperative in my recovery.
- Becoming an advocate for other victims and survivors. Being a voice for others and helping to make a change, however small, helps my recovery greatly. And I now hope to be able to develop research to help support those who experience sexual violence.
- And lastly, I followed the guidance of those who offered me advice. I listened to doctors, the gardaí, my counsellor, lecturers, family, partner and friends. I learned to trust them and their advice and unconsciously followed their guidance. That trust got me to where I am today.

My trauma still affects me, and recovery is not a destination, it is a journey. It does not mean being free from the effects of trauma, but more the ability to live a more wholesome life with it. I sometimes continue to feel lonely in my trauma but in recovery, I feel supported. To date, I continue to think about what happened to me daily, but it no longer controls me. Sometimes I regress, sometimes I leap forward. But I am kind to myself and try to accept where I am, even on my worst days. I am back in counselling once again and am happy to be. I hope to share my story more, talk more and help more. Recovery should be shared.

References

Irish Legal News. (2021). *Rape crisis charity calls for independent legal representation for victims.* https://www.irishlegal.com/articles/rape-crisis-charity-calls-for-independent-legal-representation-for-victims

McGee, H. M. (2002). *The SAVI report: Sexual abuse and violence in Ireland.* https://www.drcc.ie/assets/files/pdf/drcc_2002_savi_report_2002.pdf

Miller, A. (1981). *The drama of the gifted child: The search for the true self translated by Ruth Ward.* Harper Collins.

Recorded Crime Q4 2017. (2018, June 27). *CSO – Central Statistics Office.* https://www.cso.ie/en/releasesandpublications/ep/p-rc/recordedcrimeq42017/

Vallières, F., Gilmore, B., Nolan, A., Maguire, P., Bondjers, K., McBride, O., Murphy, J., Shevlin, M., Karatzias, T., & Hyland, P. (2020). Sexual violence and its associated psychosocial effects in Ireland. *Journal of Interpersonal Violence, 37*(11–12), NP9066–NP9088. https://doi.org/10.1177/0886260520978193

Chapter 9

Love

The Eternal Student

I am a person no better or no worse than anyone else.

I grew up on a farm in rural Ireland in a good family and for the majority, had a happy childhood and teenage years. I enjoyed helping out on the farm when I was young I was bullied in my teenage years but I had great friends in both national school and secondary school. Then I went to college and lived away from home. In college, I was bullied and ostracised by my housemates. The bullying and ostracisation encouraged me to loathe myself and lose confidence, I also chose to feel hatred for the people who bullied me.

One night when I was going to bed, I heard three people talking through the wall, two aggressive men, and a woman, trying to threaten to come into the house and attack me. I couldn't sleep all night because of the voices. I went to work and my dread, the three voices/people followed me insulting me and threatening me. The voices impacted my ability to do my job and I was overcome with fear for the entire workday. My boss and co-workers were aware of this and my boss told me I could go home early. I walked to a nearby lake and cried as the voices tormented me. Luckily, I went home to the farm. I tried challenging and running after the people that I believed were there (I didn't know then that they were voices). After days of this, I was burnt out. I remember I shared a bedroom with my younger brother. One night I said there were three people in a car, I could hear the car, I had really good hearing they were going to come into the room and attack me. My brother told me to get into the other bed in the room with him and put his arms around me and said if they come into the house we will fight them. My brother's words filled me with love and courage. Looking back now I know my brother knew there was nobody outside in the car.

My family was worried about me because I couldn't concentrate and I was hearing voices. The voices were saying that they were going to come in and attack me. They brought me to a doctor who arranged for me to see a psychiatric team. The psychiatrist asked me if I wanted to have some time to rest and I agreed.

Different Diagnoses, Similar Experiences:
Narratives of Mental Health, Addiction Recovery and Dual Diagnosis, 85–87
Published under exclusive licence by Emerald Publishing Limited
doi:10.1108/978-1-80455-848-520241009

I went to a small psychiatric unit. I was in my room and I heard the voices and began to question how the people following me didn't need to sleep, use the toilet, work or rest. How could they follow me all day long and not get tired of talking constantly? The defining moment happened when I walked from one side of the hospital to the other. How could they run around the building so quickly and talk to me from the other side of the building? Pretty soon after that, I met my psychiatrist and I told her I didn't think the voices were real, she said I was the quickest person she met to realise this. Shortly after that, I was put on a medication that took a month to work but it took away the voices.

I worked and went to college and studied and practised Buddhism. Buddhism taught me how to gain more control over my mind by putting in positive thoughts and emotions. The biggest lesson I learned from Buddhism is to try to help others (Love) this makes both them and you happy. This lesson greatly helped my recovery. I asked to have my medication changed and consequently, they changed it. After a time, the voices came back harsher and more critical than ever. I know they were just voices and not people but the voices were calling me a rapist and a paedophile and criticising me day and night. I asked a psychiatrist to put me back on the last medication that worked but they refused. They told me I changed medications too often and I had been complaining of tiredness. I went to my doctor seeking a private psychiatrist but he said the public system was the best and refused to give me the number of a private psychiatrist I tried but I couldn't find a private psychiatrist near me.

I was heavily medicated which made it hard for me to think, and worse still I was hearing critical voices. I kept at my degree, and with support from a good lecturer and fellow student, I achieved a degree in Theology and Business. I continued to work after the degree and I could still hear both critical internal and external voices. A psychiatrist informed me *'you're going to get anxiety and depression from these voices'*, in a way he was right. I had suicidal thoughts and intense anxiety around people, however with the support of a good therapist and my Buddhist teacher (B.W.), I fought the feelings of depression, social anxiety, and self-hatred. Buddhism had given me something to live for, which was to make a difference in people's lives.

It was after this my mum showed me a leaflet for a local trialogue meeting, which is a community mental health group/forum. It is very inclusive where people who use the services, people who work in the services, family members of those who are experiencing distress or recovery and those with an interest in mental wellbeing come together to discuss their experiences. I went with my brother to a place where a friend told me to talk to this person who hears voices but has recovered (P.M.). I told (P.M.) I had schizophrenia and he gave me advice on how to deal with the voices. He advised me to just talk with them tell them to go away for a while and that you will talk to them later, and dedicate them time to talk to you for an hour at night. The technique he recommended worked for months. I would talk to the voices and ask them to go away and I talked to them later to my surprise they said yes, and sometimes they would come back but I would be firm with them and ask them to go away and that I would talk to them later. (P.M.) for free had given me advice that worked that no highly paid psychiatrist had ever given me. Now I felt more in control of my voices and because they were going away I had peace of mind. (P.M.) taught me to accept and talk with the voices, and consequently, when I started to talk to the voices and give them time to talk to me I didn't feel as much of a victim. From books on voice-hearing, (P.M.) recommended, I learned that sometimes the voices represented people I know. One day I told the voices '*I love you*' and to my surprise, I heard them say back '*I love you too*'. These techniques worked for a while, talking to others about what the voices are saying to you, not being afraid of them or believing them all the time, and having an open accepting playful attitude towards the voices worked well for me There are groups where you can get help with voices, called the hearing voices network. Later (P.M.) and (L.M.) trained me as a peer support worker where I learned a lot about recovery and mental health. A peer support worker is someone who uses their own personal experience of emotional distress and recovery to support and empower the people they are supporting. Peer support has really helped my recovery. There's great joy in being a peer. It gives me an opportunity to strive to be authentic with people. Providing an empathic ear towards people's problems and accepting them unconditionally. I'm far from being perfect but I am trying to better my life and support others in recovery. It has been really good for my recovery to work with and spend time with so many good people such as peer support workers, family peers and others who use their lived experience of helping others.

It took years but eventually, the voices have got less and less. I have been taken off two medications completely, and I am reducing the third medication now. I'm lucky, with my voices as now and again they tell me jokes I enjoy the voices now. They make me laugh. I've been working as a peer support worker where I pass on the support (Love) of my brother, meditation teacher, therapist, lecturer, classmates, (P.M.) and (L.M.), and the advice (P.M.) gave me how to deal with the voices. To anybody whose struggling, especially with voices, don't hide away. Get help. There are many good people out there. I would also recommend seeking out the support of a peer support worker. There are peer support workers available in both the Health Service Executive and in the community and don't forget the hearing voices group.

Chapter 10

Transforming Torment

Andrew C. Grundy

University of Manchester, UK

In this chapter, I want to share my experiences of '*the Men*' and how they have shaped my life, both negatively, but also positively. They have brought me low, bringing psychiatric hospital admissions, but have also opened doors of opportunity for me, particularly in mental health research.

Introducing '*the Men*' – Torment and Torture

In February 2007, I started hearing terrifying noises – it was initially like someone angrily shushing me. The noises soon turned into short and sharp voices telling me to '*Shut up!*' That then turned into voices telling me how useless I was, how I should end my life etc. I could not understand what was happening to me. My GP put it down to stress – our first child had been born in November 2005 and my wife was pregnant again, I was finishing an MPhil, was trying to work too, had church responsibilities, and some dear friends had recently left the country. As I had had periods of depression in the past, I was again prescribed an antidepressant. However, the voices caused me so much distress that we eventually sought hospital admission via psychiatric liaison at A&E. I had a short admission to a psychiatric assessment ward, and they upped the dose of the antidepressant.

Then in July, just two weeks after the birth of our second child, I started hearing and seeing quite distinctly three evil men ('*the Men*') – the voices were now embodied. They were real (I lost '*insight*'). Everywhere I went they seemed to be there – there was no escaping them. They were deriding me, tormenting me, sometimes screaming and shouting and swearing at me. They started performing experiments on me – they implanted maggot-like eggs in my brain, I could feel them hatching, and the alien creatures feasting on my brain. They implanted a microchip in my hand in an attempt to try and control me – sending electric shocks up my arm when I didn't do their bidding. They, and those working for them, were trying to steal my thoughts, making me confused and forgetful. The men were also trying to insert their thoughts into my mind. They started to command me to harm some

Different Diagnoses, Similar Experiences:
Narratives of Mental Health, Addiction Recovery and Dual Diagnosis, 89–94
Copyright © 2024 by Andrew C. Grundy
Published under exclusive licence by Emerald Publishing Limited
doi:10.1108/978-1-80455-848-520241010

of those around me. They felt like all-powerful, all-knowing and godlike malevolent presences. I was utterly terrified at the thought that I might comply with their demands. I had a four-week hospital admission to a psychiatric treatment ward, during which they put me on an antipsychotic, gradually upping the dose.

That November, the same pattern – hearing the men, seeing the men, and feeling their experiments, although much more intensely and overwhelmingly. This time a three-month hospital admission. Things were getting worse, not better. My wife was told this was '*paranoid schizophrenia.*' As three antipsychotics had had no long-lasting effects, I was put on clozapine. These admissions did provide me with a certain sense of safety, in that I was away from the people that the men wanted me to harm, and away from the means to do so or to harm myself, which did reassure me. Staff seemed very interested in the form of the experiences (external or internal voices; first or third-person speech, etc.), but only really interested in certain parts of their content (for symptom severity and assessing risk). I kept having to go over my story with different staff members, thinking that I would eventually get some therapy, but that never came. Essentially, staff were using PRN, waiting for the antipsychotic to kick in and advising distraction techniques.

At this point, I want to acknowledge three constant sources of support that have been helpful to me. First, my loving wife – mercifully, whilst I doubted the loyalty of nearly everyone around me, I never doubted her. I always knew that she was on my side, working with me, against the men. Second, our amazing church family. Our church showed their love to my wife, kids, and me in very practical ways – I was never without a visitor whilst on the wards, people cooked meals, helped around the house and babysat when my wife came to visit. Whilst she received very little support from mental health services, our church stepped up and stepped in. Third, is my own Christian faith, which is a source of hope and help for me even at the darkest times; whilst there were times when I wondered whether this was the kind of life worth living, I was able to bring my despair to God. I am so thankful for these constant supports.

Beginning to Understand '*the Men*'

When I was discharged from the hospital on Valentine's Day February 2008, I was allocated a Care Coordinator (Sarah) under the Early Intervention in Psychosis team, and a Consultant Psychiatrist (Dr J.). Together, Sarah, Dr J., my wife, and I drew up a care plan, and an advanced statement of my wishes should I relapse, all of which was helpful and was reviewed annually. Between 2008 and 2010, I had a number of psychotic episodes ranging from 12 to 2 weeks, and of different severity, but with Sarah's support, I managed to stay out of hospital. Sarah then moved on, but I was allocated a new Care Coordinator (Chris), who was equally helpful and supportive.

Up until this point, my main coping strategy was distraction techniques – the unspoken message seemed to be that listening to the men would be a bad idea and that their voices needed drowning out somehow. For me, distraction involves listening to loud music on headphones, but there are limits as to how much time you can spend doing that! During this time, Sarah introduced me to the *Hearing Voices Network*. I joined a local mental health day centre, which had a small hearing voices group. It was helpful being around others with similar experiences to my own. My wife started reading books by Marius Romme and Sandra Escher, and she started passing on the key messages to me – which opened my eyes to a new means of engaging with voices.

At this stage, the key step we took was to try to understand the men, to build up a character profile of each of them, by starting to listen to them intentionally and asking them questions. I then began to transcribe some of the conversations. These transcripts would become significant for me in therapy later, but for now, the increased understanding made me realise that they often said things that were simply untrue (they weren't all-knowing), and that they often made threats that they did not follow through on (they weren't all-powerful). Increasingly, I felt able, at times, to say back to them '*I don't believe you!*' All this began to make me feel less fearful of them. We also read about negotiation and bargaining – I began asking the men that if I gave them some protected time, promising to listen and transcribe what they had to say, would they, for example, give me sleep that night. That often worked, and again gave me a real feeling of empowerment and a sense of regaining control over my life.

Exploiting '*the Men*'

Getting into Research

In November 2010, I was approached by a keyworker at the day centre with a flyer. It was an advert for a training course in research methods for service users and carers being run by a team of researchers. I wasn't sure it would be interesting or beneficial to me, but they were paying people to attend, so I went for it! I was interviewed for the opportunity that December and was then invited to join the training course, for one day a month, January – June 2011, up at Manchester University. The course covered an introduction to study skills, qualitative methods, quantitative methods, critical appraisal of research papers, ethics and dissemination.

The course was part of a programme development grant to train up service users and carers to become involved in a full programme grant. I was then invited to join the study team as a co-applicant and co-investigator on the research programme that would become 'EQUIP: Enhancing the quality of service user-involved care planning in mental health services'. The research programme ran from September 2012 to September 2016. For the role, I was employed as a part-time Research Associate at the University of Nottingham in February 2013 and stayed in that post until September 2016.

Over time, I began to realise that my experiences of '*the Men*' (my experience of mental distress, of services, treatments, professionals, processes, etc.) were being treated like credentials, like a form of knowledge and expertise. What I had only thought of as deficits were now being turned into assets, and that I could use some of the darkest moments of my life to make a difference. I realised that the researchers who only had a learned knowledge of the topic were looking for wisdom and insight from those who had lived experience of it. I felt like I was making an impact on the research, but this also had a positive and empowering impact on me.

Being involved in EQUIP was good for me for a number of other reasons. It satisfied my intellectual curiosity that had laid dormant during the difficult days, I was constantly learning new things and developing new skills. It was good to build new relationships with people and to feel part of a team. It was helpful to be in employment, which gave us some financial stability as a family, and I appreciated the ability to work part-time and flexitime. I also felt that the focus of the research I was involved in could make a real difference to other service users. I think there was also a sense of giving something back to services.

Adjusting to a New Way of Life

At the same time as all this was happening, in early 2012 I was transferred from the Early Intervention service to the Community Mental Health Team. Thankfully, I stayed under Dr J, and we really appreciated that continuity. The main source of support was now my monthly check-in at the clozapine clinic. I decided that I wanted to rely more on the psychological techniques I had learned than medication. Whilst my consultant expressed some concerns, she was supportive of my decision to gradually reduce the dose. In April 2013, I had a sudden 'red' blood test warning, and I was told that I had to come off the medication immediately. Long story short, I had clozapine withdrawal syndrome, ended up in hospital on a neurological ward following some non-epileptic seizures, and had a short, rebound psychotic episode. However, at this point, I was determined to try and stay off antipsychotics altogether.

I continued in my research role – but it had its difficulties. I found performance reviews stressful as I didn't feel like I was a '*real*' researcher. I wasn't well prepared for the emotional labour of research. I found trying to fit lots of interviews into a tight timeframe emotionally draining and difficult, and struggled with time management. Quite unexpectedly, I found interviewing some of the carers really challenging – they were often sharing how emotionally difficult it was supporting their family member, and I was left feeling upset and that I was a massive burden on my own wife and children. This triggered a psychotic episode and a four-week period of hospitalisation in November 2013, just as I had finished all my interviews.

During this admission, my new way of working with the men also came under fire – the consultant said he had never heard of voice dialogue before, and with me being very reluctant to go back on antipsychotics, we didn't have a great therapeutic relationship. I was desperately looking for someone who could simply sit with me and support me whilst I engaged with the men – but staff were concerned, because they didn't know whether this was clinically helpful or not. In the end, we got around the impasse, as I was referred to inpatient psychological services. The clinical psychologist that I saw during the admission endorsed my coping strategies, but he raised the idea that a short-term return to antipsychotics might give me the strength and stability to do more of the psychological work. I went back on an antipsychotic, but only to serve that purpose.

I was again dealing with the usual fear of the men, but I was also worried that the staff thought I was working undercover, researching their own care planning processes! This time I knew that I should be involved in my care planning, and I wanted to contribute to my care plan. I simply wanted to write '*I am being tormented by three evil men who are conducting experiments on me*' – but a senior nurse informed me that I couldn't do that, as they were not prepared to '*collude with my delusions*'. At the same time, I was able to talk to the nurses in training about the importance of good and service user-involved care planning!

I went back to EQUIP in January 2014, with monthly supervision arrangements in place, which made a real difference. I was also allocated a Care Coordinator (Kate) under the Community Mental Health Team, who was a really good source of support. I was able to process with her some of the stigmas I was facing – some from friends (my wife was asked if she felt safe around me), some from the news (I felt shame at every mass shooting, where suddenly there was speculation about the perpetrator's mental state). It made me not want to be open, and not want to seek further help – but it was good to talk with her about it.

That April, I experienced another psychotic episode. I tried to show the Crisis Team staff that I could cope using only my voice dialogue techniques, but I just couldn't focus enough to transcribe anything and got completely overwhelmed. They recommended another admission, and I had another four weeks in hospital. This time I felt coerced back onto clozapine, with the consultant basically saying that they could use the Mental Health Act unless I complied. Once I was stabilised on the clozapine, I was discharged. However, a condition of discharge this time around was that I would be referred for support from Outpatient Psychological Services.

After a wait of 16 months(!) that felt like an age, I got to see a clinical psychologist. We started to talk about a number of things. We talked about my past trauma. We also explored some of the key themes that came out of my transcripts of conversations with the men that I had kept. I started to see that, for me, it seemed to make sense that these experiences were projections of my past trauma. And that the men were saying things that deep down I believed about myself. The men had, in effect, identified the issues to be talked through in therapy. It was also helpful for me to acknowledge how traumatising it had been to have these experiences – essentially being verbally and emotionally abused and even physically tortured (the experiments and electric shocks), by the men over so many periods of time. And it was good too to talk about how they had had a massive impact on my sense of self – my self-esteem, my self-confidence and my self-compassion. I couldn't understand why I'd never had this kind of support before, but it was enormously helpful. I think I really dealt with the past. It helped give me a deeper sense of stability.

Onto a Career?

By the time the EQUIP programme came to an end, I felt I had enough stability to do something in research full-time. I had always wanted to do a PhD, and the opportunity came up to apply for a scholarship from the School of Health

Sciences at the University of Nottingham. Being awarded this was a massive confidence boost and in September 2016 I embarked on the PhD programme. I knew that I wanted to focus on risk assessment and management in mental health and on psychiatric inpatient care in particular. I had experienced this as covert, disempowering, and traumatising and wanted to see how other service users had experienced this. Turns out, there wasn't much evidence out there. I conducted my study on one acute inpatient ward – it felt weird going back onto a ward, but thankfully, with good supervision, it wasn't triggering for me. I should probably write elsewhere about all the issues around doing this kind of research as a lived experience researcher, because it raised so many issues for me. I was so thankful to my participants, and I hope my thesis did them justice. The whole PhD took me five years.

At the age of 46, I do now feel like I've now started a career. After I finished my PhD, in November 2021, I began mainly working as a Lived Experience Researcher at the University of Manchester. At the time of writing, I am working on a project called SUSTAIN, which is looking at helping service users to manage the hunger side-effects of antipsychotics. My other job role is that I am currently working as the Lived Experience Research Lead at the Mental Health Policy Research Unit, UCL, for two days a week. These roles all include working with other people with lived experience, helping to involve and include them in research projects, and training and mentoring them. The roles also involve training academic staff in involvement and co-production, with strategic oversight of that in the organisations.

Reflections on Coping with '*the Men*'

I am now in a completely different stage of life than when I first entered mental health services back in 2007. I have greatly benefitted from my family and community support networks – I realise that many people don't have that kind of help and support, and I don't think I'd be where I am now without them. I have my faith, which is an enormous comfort and source of hope for me. I have found ways of managing my distress that have helped me – I have benefitted at times from medication, but I have benefitted more from voice dialogue. I recognise that the episodic nature of my psychosis means that I have periods of stability when I am really well – which have, mercifully, increased over time. I have been able to do a job that gives me satisfaction and meaning, and I can even use my lived experience in it to make a difference. I have had Care Coordinators and a community Consultant who I've had good relationships with, who have honoured my decisions and have been willing to think outside the biomedical box. I've benefitted from formal psychological support; the outpatient therapy was particularly transformative. I'm mindful that whilst I'm on an even path now, it could only take a big life-changing event to knock me down again. I don't know if I'll ever see the men again, but I'm now hopeful that I now have the skills to manage come what may.

Chapter 11

Nothing In, Nothing Out

Jenny Langley

'You never make things fun enough!' A childish comment, delivered by a child in a run of the mill childish moment. But the pin had been pulled from the grenade a few weeks earlier and I was tired of holding the explosion at bay. Even now, two years on, the abruptness of the nosedive I took that day shocks me. I was in the midst of party organising: beer bargains secured, burgers and buns procured, folding chairs put out, barbeque fired up. But apparently it wasn't enough. I wasn't enough. I would never be enough. So, I slipped away, ostensibly to calm down, though I found myself surrendering completely, pulled in by the shadows while the others took in the sun.

All afternoon, I lay watching shafts of light and shade track paths around the bedroom, listening to the kids on the road – mine among them – carousing at full force. Later, they were joined by their parents, who used the good weather as a limp excuse to meet, drink beer and make merry. The lightness and laughter of my neighbours vibrated in the air around me and ordinarily would have drawn me back to life. But inside my skin, I was already dying. And as the sun burnt itself out, I felt what little brightness there was left in me extinguish with it.

Periodically my husband came in, his anxious face peering round the door, asking me to join the gang outside. I didn't answer. It was all I could do to shake my head – a monumental effort, undertaken only because this cloister was my last safe space and I wanted it to myself. At some point that afternoon, I realised I had crawled in here because it was time to die. I lay, catatonic, waiting for my family to return and sleep, so that I could find a way to slip out of my house and their life, without them watching.

For hours, my brain churned thoughts in panicky spirals; a woolly mess that became further entangled the more I tried to tease it out. I was ashamed, confused, angry... But mostly I was just hopelessly sad. It was directed at myself, at everyone, at no one in particular. I had no idea yet how I had come to this place, or what was even real any more. There was no sense to be made from my thoughts or the emotions they elicited. One part of me eye-rolled at the melodrama; another raged savagely; another cried like a child and just wanted to be

Different Diagnoses, Similar Experiences:
Narratives of Mental Health, Addiction Recovery and Dual Diagnosis, 95–101
Copyright © 2024 by Jenny Langley
Published under exclusive licence by Emerald Publishing Limited
doi:10.1108/978-1-80455-848-520241011

held. But more and more, I thought with relief about the final step and the breeze I'd feel under my feet as I fell. I lay waiting for the world to sleep, my brain at war with itself. It was too much. It was all just too much. I was desperate to let go of it all. I wasn't even sure what 'it' was.

Finally, exhausted by the revelry, my family crept home to the dark house I feigned sleep in, and found their own peaceful slumber. Hours later, I found my way down the stairs, trying not to look at their sleeping bodies.

It seems nonsensical now, but my plans were undone by a pair of missing shoes and I find that strangely embarrassing to admit. I couldn't face the several miles of cut feet I'd have to endure without them, but was afraid to go back upstairs and retrieve them, and quite honestly, the realisation that other shoes were likely nearby escaped me. I stood, stricken, in the middle of the kitchen, incapable of finding a solution. I've described this moment to a friend before. She called it an 'epiphany of stasis'. There is such poignant accuracy in that phrase. Somewhere outside my range of conscious thought, I think the organism I walk around in wanted to survive, so it incapacitated me.

Instead, the remainder of the night was spent lying on the couch, crying: my body unmoving, still wearing the previous day's clothes and the dried-in kisses of my children. As the hours passed, I begged silently to be found, to not be found, to be saved, to die. I was afraid to move, because I'd be stepping towards death. I was afraid to stay still because to do so would mean to live another day. There was just terror, confusion and precisely zero hope.

I passed out just as the sun came up and Jonny found me a short time later, sending me gently back to bed. I don't know when he began to worry, but by the end of my second day lying in the same position, on the same bed, staring at the same tree, out the same window, still refusing to speak, eat, drink, move, engage... By that stage, he was concerned about my state of mind and somewhere in the background, outside my range of awareness and he began to seek out my allies.

I can see that over the course of that second day, thoughts of my family were taking root. Little tendrils of resistance and reaching out for a reason to stay. There was still solace in imagining that final step and taking flight into fresh air. The sweet relief it would bring. But, I'd known the loss of a parent while still in school myself and the realisation of what I'd be doing to my own family cut me deeply. My kids would look for someone to curl into for comfort and no one else would fit the same way. Jonny would lose his best friend and strongest ally. My mum would have to live with the ache of a missing child – something I cata-strophised about myself.

As the battle continued to rage in me, a mantra formed itself in my lungs. My incantation for survival: 'nothing in, nothing out'. I continued to lie, unmov-ing, simply breathing, refusing to speak or consume anything other than oxygen. Two more days, I repeated it. Nothing in, nothing out. I breathed in and held on to life. I breathed out and let go of it. And so it continued, until the love of my family, the care of my doctor and the guidance of staff in A&E carried me to the safety of a psychiatric ward.

This is the point in the story where you might expect the carnage trope to kick in; panic, loneliness, prison-like conditions, the indignity of queuing for medication and the boredom of hour after hour of nothing happening. You won't read that from me. I spent ten glorious weeks in the hospital and treasure each one of them. I needed the space and the time, the quiet and the permission to do nothing. I needed to be cut off from the outside world so that I could filter out the noise and distraction and begin to listen inwards again.

Not that I liked what I heard in there. Not at all.

A few caveats: I was not in a locked ward; I was not in psychosis; mine was a voluntary admission; and, I had private health insurance. All of those things, based on what I've learnt since, impacted hugely on my experience as a psychiatric patient.

Psychiatric patient. There is something resistant in me when I see, hear or read that term. *Me?* A psychiatric patient? Doesn't that imply that I'm ill in some way? Sick in the head? It doesn't feel like me. I really don't feel like it applies. Even then it didn't feel like it 'fit'. I was just sad, lost, confused, hurt, lonely and utterly, utterly devoid of hope.

The first days of my new reality were terrifying. My belongings were searched and several items were withheld for my own safety. The demeanour of other patients on the ward was often confusing, and the behaviour of some was alarming. I felt completely alone, out of my depth and had no idea at all what to expect. It didn't help that I was admitted over a Bank Holiday weekend and had to wait several days to meet my consultant. By the time that happened, however, I'd been moved to a quieter ward, where I could finally unpack my belongings and start to feel a little more at home.

Still, my mantra held: Nothing In, Nothing Out. I could not eat. I barely spoke. But I took every pill they handed me, grateful for the numbness they afforded by day and the oblivion of sleep they facilitated each night. I avoided contact with the outside world, ashamed of the state I'd fallen into and the burden I was placing on those who loved me most. Desperate for some peace and anonymity.

I cried a lot. Thinking of my children asking where I was made me cry. Thinking of my mum as she lay on the bed trying to reach me and stroking my hair made me cry. Believing I was turning into my husband's worst nightmare made me cry. Fathoming how I'd ended up in this facility made me cry. Wondering how, or when, or *if*, I could ever safely leave this place made me cry. The fear that I might never feel like a whole human again made me cry. I was infected generally with an 'insidious pus of fear', as my wonderful, articulate friend might say.

Days eked by, meds kicked in and the quiet began to take over. I met people, lovely people; strange, sick, troubled, crazy people who felt, like me, that something fundamental had been broken in them. And as the weeks rolled round and I found solace in there, I began to cherish my place in this band of misfits. I felt at home with the other crazies and began to see their 'illnesses', and mine, in a different light. Our brains were not sick, our spirits were simply broken.

It was enlightening to realise that all of us – whether we were depressed, addicted, bipolar or psychotic – all had something in common. Trauma. We were all struggling to survive in the wake of something or things that had irrevocably damaged us. Now, I've learned enough to realise that just as our DNA and the minutiae of our life stories are unique to each of us, so is our response to the vagaries of the lives we live. Things happen and we adapt to them, we develop coping strategies to help keep our heads above water. For some that's obsessive behaviours and routines; for others its voices that no one else can hear; for others still it's cutting the skin to let the pain out; for me, it was imagining myself ending everything and knowing that there was always a way out if I couldn't keep going. Psychiatry views these things as 'symptoms', manifestations of 'illness'. The rest of the world considers them proof that we're crazy. To those of us experiencing them, they are survival tactics, a means of processing our reality, maintaining control and *staying sane*. Slowly, I started to become aware that what the rest of the world thinks of as mental illness is actually just a 'normal reaction to a set of abnormal circumstances'.

My mantra held, the whole ten weeks through. Its nuance shifted though. As the stranglehold, I felt trapped in began to loosen, and I started to feel less threatened, the realisation dawned that I'd only get out what I put into the experience: 'nothing in, nothing out!' This time was an investment in myself and my future wellbeing. This was an opportunity to right some wrongs and begin the process of rebuilding myself, of healing.

So, I took up yoga. I journaled. I went to mindfulness sessions and took a CBT course. I ate well, slept like a hero, took my meds religiously and exercised constantly. And gradually, I began to emerge back into the world, taking hours out from the hospital to shop, or visit family, or walk the pier in Dun Laoghaire.

Early one morning, I left the hospital to bring my daughter to her first day of Junior Infant, but quickly realised I was out of my depth. Too soon. Surrounded by people from before, who knew nothing of what was going on behind the scenes, the brief immersion in normality terrified me, and I realised I was not yet functional enough for the world. I scurried back to the hospital, with a renewed awareness of my vulnerability and an intensified terror at the prospect of leaving the hospital for good.

The hospital wasn't all communing with nature and namaste. There were really tough parts. Some of the sessions I had with psychologists and social workers were excruciating. I had to face up to the damage caused to me by two serious sexual assaults – one as a child and one in my twenties. Then began the process of examining the wounds they had caused and the impact they'd had on my life and relationships. The toughest part was learning to say the word 'rape' out loud, in relation to myself. Even now, that word feels hard and dangerous in my mouth, like vomiting up a mouthful of nails. My social worker helped me to disclose these experiences to my mother and husband safely, and later, helped me to report them to Gardai.

Much as I recognised and appreciated the shelter and respite the hospital afforded me, there were elements of the experience that I found troubling. On arriving at my first MDT meeting (Multi-Disciplinary Team), I found myself – already in a distressed and dishevelled state – facing a room full of power-dressed mental health professionals, apparently gathered en masse to facilitate the best possible response to my 'illness'. But let me tell you: sitting alone, facing a panel which incorporated a psychiatrist, psychologist, social worker, pharmacist, occupational therapist, a couple of registrars and at least two nurses – none of whom

I'd ever met before – was one of the most humiliating experiences of my life. They call it 'person-centred', but it felt 'patient-focused', a subtle but important difference. They all looked so put-together, so *im*personal and *un*approachable. I thought this space was meant to be safe. Every time I spoke someone tap-tapped each of my words into a computer. They sat, silent and observant, while I tried not to fidget or cry. The psychiatrist addressed me, and I him. The others rarely spoke, and when they did so, they often reacted as if caught in a spotlight, challenged and uncomfortable. I wondered how many of them realised that I felt the exact same way. Twice a week for the duration of my stay I faced down this menacing throng, and although I learned to cope with it well enough, it never once felt comfortable, reassuring or remotely helpful to be examined under the glare of so many professional gazes.

I can see now, too, that I was suffering from white-coat syndrome – believing in the sanctity of my medical team's supreme knowledge and expertise. That is dangerous, because it meant that I trusted them more than my own gut and I believe they encouraged that. When the nursing staff voiced concern that I was 'inappropriately over-engaging' with other patients, they undermined my sense of companionship and solidarity amongst my peers. When my psychiatrist told me that, 'these people are not your friends; you'll leave this hospital and never see these people again', he undermined my faith in my own ability to recognise authenticity and be safe in the relationships around me. They were all wrong, by the way. I was good at supporting my peers, they were good at supporting me and I'm still in regular contact with quite a lot of them.

Question marks aside, I'm immensely grateful for the ten weeks I had 'inside'. In fact, I frequently wish myself back there, just for a teeny stint of respite!

When I finally came home, I was still fairly rigid with apprehension. I knew that I'd only just begun the journey towards recovery, and many of the demons that frightened me were waiting just inside the front door. The overwhelming responsibility of guiding tiny humans through life was a mantle I would once more have to assume. I still tended to smooth over how things *really* were, and just say 'fine'. I had still identified no clear purpose or direction for myself, beyond the menial tasks of cleaning counters and filling the fridge. Even the ocean of Legos that drowned out my son's carpet felt too much. But the time I'd invested in learning to acknowledge and face my fears would ultimately pay off. I had put in the time, and now, I was reaping the benefits. Something in, something out.

I'm an all-or-nothing kind of person. So when I came home, I felt the need to throw myself headfirst into my recovery: I did Compassion Focused Therapy and a Wellness Recovery Action Plan course. I did yoga, continued with the gym, took my meds, did mindfulness every night and visited a psychologist regularly. I tried peer support groups online, tried to keep up journaling and read whatever I could find online about how to support my recovery. I committed myself to forward momentum. Don't stop to see how far you haven't come yet. One more step and then one more. The sense of control that gave me had a kind of placebo effect. I marched onward towards the promised land of Recovery.

Recovery, it's an interesting word, and I remember the first time I was confronted with it in the context of my mental health. We were having friends around for dinner. One of them had just been through a mental health crisis of his own, and we discussed how our respective depressive symptoms manifested. His wife and my husband compared notes on what it was like to live with people in this situation, and in attempting to draw a line under the conversation, my friend said: 'I just want to focus on my recovery'. The physicality of my reaction was visceral; I honestly felt in that moment as if I'd been punched in the face. Recovery, was a word that could never, *ever* apply to me. How could I 'get back' to being someone I'd never been, given that depression had been bounding in and out of my life for the past thirty years? Suddenly the rest of my life yawned in front of me like the blackest of stifling tunnels, with no discernible end. This was the stunning moment when the grenade pin was pulled. The street party was less than a fortnight later.

And I am weirdly thankful now, for the ensuing blowing-apart of my life, because without it, I'd never have walked into that tunnel. And as it transpired there was simply a sharp bend obscuring the exit. Nothing in, Nothing out.

It is intensely gratifying to say that recovery *is*, indeed, a word that I can claim as my own. However, my recovery was more of a re-covering. In Japan, there is a longstanding tradition, called kintsugi, of repairing broken delph by gluing the parts back together with a lacquer that is mixed with gold, silver or platinum. The idea of kintsugi is that rather than masking or hiding the cracks caused by breakage, the brokenness of the object should be cherished as part of its experience, and the cracks, chips and 'imperfections' highlighted and made beautiful, or at least imbued with meaning. That, to me, is what recovery, means. I have travelled back over my trauma, acknowledged and examined the imperfections it has created, and done my best to reframe them as something that I can cherish. Am I glad I was raped? No. Do I value the experience? No. But the lessons learnt, and the growth I have salvaged from this process of healing? That, I can treasure. Therein lies the gold fault line. And the strength.

By redressing my broken pieces in gilt-edges, my recovery has gifted me a sense of agency, a measure of self-compassion, and an awareness that my story is *mine* to tell. It is not for any medical professional to say that I am 'sick', or talk about the 'next time' that I have a crisis and 'get ill' (which has happened and much to my shock). I am not sick. I am not broken. I am not a patient with a set of symptoms. I am nothing less than a full, complex, imperfect human, with a full, complex, imperfect set of thoughts and feelings which ebb and flow more gently now that the emotional weather is more clement.

In the (almost) two years since I entered the hospital, I have discovered a compassion for myself I didn't know was possible. I have nourished it and learned to flourish from it. I have given and received help and support and authenticity from so many others in similar situations. Last September, I went back to college in order to train to become a Mental Health Peer Support Worker, and for the first time in my life (not exaggerating), I felt I had a purpose that made me happy to get out of bed in the mornings. As part of the course, I had to secure an internship/placement working with others experiencing mental distress. The peers I have worked with are, by much of society's superficial standards, not 'successful'. But they are some of the toughest, worthiest, most genuine and warmest individuals I have ever encountered. I love being a Peer Support Worker and I love the opportunity it gives me to be with people who 'get' me, and whom I can connect with in return.

Recovery (or re-covery!) is a slow, intricate and at times frustrating process, and one that is never truly complete, because – despite the gilding – you will never achieve an unblemished-as-before whole. However, the shards we break into are as unique as our DNA, and our fault lines are what we choose to make of them. So, the almost-whole you achieve will contain its own unique beauty and value. It will be what differentiates you from all those around you, and you will know that you are made almost whole by your own design and your own ability to apply care and attention, lovingly, as you craft yourself.

I have invested my full self in this process of recovery; all my pieces and all my gold. I am all in. And I am getting so much back in return.

Chapter 12

Life in the Circular Lane

Anonymous

A human following a deeply reflective life, breaking patterns, who is a jack of all trades but master of none. Deeply interested in humans and helping and learning to rest.

It's always hard to know where to begin when you are talking about trauma and diagnosis. Not to skim over a lot of it but I led a very colourful childhood. I grew up in a house that had domestic violence, psychological, physical and emotional abuse. It cascaded over us daily and while efforts were made to attempt to protect us from it, it seeped in every pore of both the house and us as individuals. It was burned into us that we do not talk or tell others and by the time I was a teenager, I was a ticking timebomb of un-navigated trauma.

I had been through multiple social workers, counsellors and court mandated appointments and by 13 I rejected them all and refused to go. I had to appear in court before a judge and write off the parent in front of said parent after spending hours waiting in the cold harsh waiting space in the courtroom beside him. These very experiences led to my Mam working with other single parents to create reform in the courthouse in Kilkenny so later families would not have to face the same thing.

For me, the damage was done. There were two uncivilised words I spent my whole life being called, one crudely describes female anatomy and the other a woman who sells her body for money. These would shape my slippery slope to mental life hell more than I knew at the time. The resultant factor was I went from an A student to a D student. I was told repeatedly that I was a drama queen and invalidated and repeatedly dismissed even by medical teams.

When I was 17 they gave me antidepressants for self-harm and suicidal ideation. I had started drinking at 14 and as I had a steady job since then had the means to supply myself with sugar and booze. I was old for my age, was not carded till my 18th birthday and as such was in freefall on a downward spiral that no one caught.

Different Diagnoses, Similar Experiences:
Narratives of Mental Health, Addiction Recovery and Dual Diagnosis, 103–106
Copyright © 2024 by Anonymous
Published under exclusive licence by Emerald Publishing Limited
doi:10.1108/978-1-80455-848-520241012

At 20 an event occurred which destroyed me. I was away on holiday when it occurred and had not even been drinking which meant the spike in my sprite doubly affected me as there was no alcohol to reduce its effects the detectives told me. I was a mess, found lying on O'Connell Street in a drunken blob, guards picked me up and put me on the Dublin Bus back over to Thomas Street where I was living at the time and where I attempted to end my life.

My next recollection is ending up in the hospital, on suicide watch in Dublin, where I lived for three months before the majority of my family and friends found out. It was a hellscape. I smoked 50 cigarettes a day, drank tea and just died inside. I was so drugged I didn't know my elbow from my proverbial and the decision was that I would relocate to the UK with my family to live with family. It would not succeed, I just drowned without support and floundered from space to space.

Then I rang my Mam for the second time in a day unusually. I was really upset and just wanted to hear her voice. I never could have imagined the chapter that phone call would open, I heard a beep in the background, one I recognised as a hospital machine, I asked where she was, she said at home watching Corrie, the machine beeped again, I called her bluff and it was then I discovered she had been unwell and in hospital for weeks. within a couple of months, we were made aware it was cancer, a few short months after that, she was dead. The same week she died, 2 other family members died and a friend of mine all passed away coincidentally and I was accused of killing my Mam by my Dad and that cemented my life spiral. Mere months after this I was engaged to a guy I had met on the way home from the UK the week of that life changing phone call. Then pregnant. I gave birth the week of all the first anniversaries and I just was not there. He broke off the engagement pre-birth. Disassociated, alone, numb to everything I sat in a realm of suicidal ideation and fighting it.

Watching that mini human gurgle at me was the reason I fought, I wanted him to grow up in a world where there was hope and where the adults around him, worked to improve life for him, not drag him into the destruction.

Now it might sound like a simple lightbulb moment, but it was far from that. I had no idea that that decision would be the easiest part of the journey. The pre-contemplation as such. I found a childminder because I was aware via therapy at this point that I was disassociated and needed that support around childcare. I wanted him to have some stability and normality. The girl I got was INCRED-IBLE. She is a vital part of the success because without her the contemplative path would not have been achieved. She charged me next to nothing and was so patient and caring both to the child and me. I was blessed with her. It meant I could finish my degree and had the support to do so! The college counsellor was also AMAZ-ING. She helped me identify my red flags by asking questions about basics every session. I learned at this point if I wasn't eating, showering etc they were pointers to me not being in a good place. This knowledge has lasted me forever since.

The preparation stage caught me once college finished and that network was gone. I was caught in a vicious loop of pre-contemplation to preparation. I will say this much in hindsight, while I would get defeated and crash, I never gave up. I moved several times during this stage for different reasons and eventually met an incredible soul who loved me as a friend despite my flaws. Her love supported me to finally break that cycle and I moved onto the action stage for the first time successfully. I did really well for a while however I was not in a holistic support space meaning that despite the success the all-round supports were not available.

It meant that when another event occurred, one in which I thought I was going to actually die that the spiral was savage and full. I was not even in precontemplation stage at this point. I ran. Moved away from the place it had occurred and despite doing everything recommended by the authorities the person was not brought to justice. It was also a wake-up call. It was 2015. I thought it was the end. So, I returned to my hometown after a brief time living by the seaside to restore my soul.

Here I leaned into all the supports, medical, mental and otherwise. We discovered I was highly functioning with severely chronic depression and anxiety, I was diagnosed with PTSD[1] and later C-PTSD[2] along with B.E.D.[3] I felt validation after years of just being labelled a drama queen. I returned to work that had been a passion of mine. The man who took me in was a vital part of changing my life and preparing me for the future where I would live and not just exist. He nurtured my creative talent. Believed in me when I couldn't believe in myself and he was the reason I could eat on some of my toughest financial days as he provided snacks for work. It was here a couple of years later I met a guy who was being interviewed who literally changed my life. We chatted, and it got deeper, he listened, didn't scoff and listened more. The first male who had not hurt or invalidated me outside of this safe space of work. He made suggestions about other supports that I had never heard of. I went and took a chance on these suggestions and I learned more about behaviour and myself.

I took the learnings and invested them into myself. I made it round the circle fully, finally. I grew and branched out in work and was never afraid to ask for help again sometimes eventually. I have since relapsed many times but never to the extent of before. This time I knew there were people around me to help and people who would listen when I was ready to speak. The valleys are super deep sometimes and they are hard as I have to fight the intrusive thoughts. I did extensive therapy on myself because I realised shame and guilt were drowning me quicker than any event was. I like to use the analogy of a heart machine recorder for my life. Those peaks are like no one other, the contentment and celebration of all the work that has led to this point. Those valleys require me to fight minute by minute or daily sometimes and they are dark and unforgiving but there are moments of balance on the incline and descent. One thing it will never be is 'just balanced' because that would be a flat line and on a heart monitor if there is a flat line, you are dead. I associate that 'death' persay to dissociation. Being here but being so numb to here that there is no 'here'.

In recovery, for me, maintenance is not just a stage in a cycle, it is life. It is learning about myself so intricately that the red flags, flag themselves to my

---

[1]Post-Traumatic Stress Disorder
[2]Complex Post-Traumatic Stress Disorder
[3]Binge Eating Disorder

consciousness. Sometimes it's quicker than others. Recovery has mainly been about learning boundaries and what I do and do not accept. This has been the toughest. When you are not sure of yourself and looking for validation, I have found that you make choices to please people in order to feel like you are accepted. Sometimes, no matter what you do, people will take advantage of you and it can impede your recovery. Sometimes you can impede others. People are mostly doing their best and it can be misguided sometimes. Other times people are taking advantage. Part of the journey is navigating who is who.

This lesson saw me step back from all the areas in my life in order to really figure out where my boundaries were and how to best progress with this new version of me. I am not impervious to anything I have learned thanks to recovery and it has led me to a great deal of understanding as life has crept up on me with various lessons. I am the child of two people who met at alcoholics anonymous and I refuse to let the same circumstances which consumed my parents consume my child. I continue to be labelled and sectioned into various types of brackets. None of that matters to me. It's all about communication and community. Without those two massive factors, I would not be here and my child and I would be another statistic. All of this is deeply personal and does not belittle someone who made a choice that I fight against or who does not believe what I do. Recovery I have learned is so individual that it's hard to write about for fear of invalidating someone else's experience. Learning from the people I have, I trust that my journey is my own and all I can ever share is that experience.

Part 3

Addiction

Chapter 13

My Name Is Paul...

Paul

My name is Paul, and I am 58 years of age and have suffered from addiction issues for over 4 decades. I am writing this now almost two years back in recovery after a series of grim relapses after a five-year period of being substance-free. I can, hand on heart say that I have rarely felt so grounded as I do right now and am blessed with many wonderful things happening in my life. This writing is more of a reflective piece rather than a war story. I have many people and agencies to be grateful for, to be at the stage where I feel hopeful, positive and in a good state of mind. To frame my thoughts around this attempt to put some parts of my life down on paper I need to be mindful of the fact that this is neither a plea for recognition nor a tale of bitterness, my story is just another version of any addict's attempt to live in the world with a mind that tries to sabotage the positive things in our life at every turn. It's my story yes, but has many similarities with so many of my peers in recovery and indeed, that identification is where I draw my strength for the most part. I don't think anyone sets out to become an addict, yet a great many people are addicted to behaviours, work, shopping, porn, food and of course substances to soothe some internal need, fear, or trauma. I am further aware that some of the people I love may read this also and so will try to just be as honest as I can while being mindful to avoid any hurt to anyone.

Early Days

When I look back on my early years it's hard to see where my addiction thinking (because that's all it is at the beginning) began but I certainly displayed some of the character traits that are relevant to people with addiction issues like a sense of aloneness, a desire to seek out that state and find comfort in isolation. I was a bit of a daydreamer as a child and an avid reader from the time I could read my own books. It has to be said that I did not grow up in a chaotic household, with no abuse or violence and neither of my parents was in addiction (at that time), my mother in later years lost her own battle with addiction. I was the second eldest of four siblings and grew up in a middle-class area in Dublin. We were brought

Different Diagnoses, Similar Experiences:
Narratives of Mental Health, Addiction Recovery and Dual Diagnosis, 109–115
Copyright © 2024 by Paul
Published under exclusive licence by Emerald Publishing Limited
doi:10.1108/978-1-80455-848-520241013

up to respect hard work and the benefits that come with that, both my folks were decent working-class people who wanted a better life for us all as a family. My mother ran the household with a firm grip, and she set a budget which enabled three of us to attend private schools. My dad was a plasterer and worked hard for the quality of life we enjoyed. As it turned out, only three of us managed to finish school and all three went on to become addicts and mess up our lives. My poor dad could never get his around what had gone awry with us.

We always had what we needed and not necessarily what we wanted; my mother was adamant about that. In fairness to her, she showed her love for us in a no-nonsense approach to keeping a clean, well-organised home, clean clothes, and food on the table every evening. She was tough and somewhat aloof, but she was there for us in her own way. My first memory of anything negative was that first day at school at the age of four, I don't think I fully understood that to be in school was not to have, for the first time, my mother nearby. In those days, the Christian Brother schools were grim, dark, and full of religious iconography and statues. Scary, to me anyway. I pretty much hated and was frightened of school as I went forward. It was not a place for softness or neediness, and I found it difficult at first.

Growing Up

As I grew up, I became incredibly adaptable in slotting into whatever situation I happened to be in but, although I may not have shown it outwardly I was quite a scared little kid and to this day don't fully understand why. Within the family dynamic, I was a 'good' child and went along with whatever was expected of me but was genuinely happier on my own. Apart from my sister, I could quite contentedly go without interaction from those around me. The first feeling of well-being I clung to was reading, particularly folk tales, fantasy and the like. This total immersion in stories and fantasy was the first sign of my predisposition to escape into another world. Now, in recovery, I am doing my best to recover from a lifetime of trying to escape reality in one way or another, avoiding responsibility, feelings and emotions became my default position in life. I don't know why I came to have that need to be cushioned from life but at the age of twelve when I took my first drink and later that year my first use of drugs my future was well and truly mapped out. I absolutely loved the effect that drugs (and I include alcohol in that) had on me, they seemed to make me feel whole and less afraid and bolstered my self-esteem. As I went through school, I looked forward to the weekends to hang out with mates who, like me, liked to get totally wasted. I never, from the word go, had a sense of moderation or self-control when using any form of substance.

Dependence

Something in me was instantly responsive to the effect of drugs, ever eager to indulge as often as possible. As I progressed through my teenage years, so too, did my experimentation and use of different drugs progress. During the last few years of school and on into my training in the hospitality sector, I was a habitual user and would be using one or more drugs throughout the day. In my career, alcohol and other drugs were just a part of the working day and that just ramped up at the end of every shift so between the circle of friends I had and my work colleagues, using was just what we did, and I fitted into this lifestyle easily. I fell for stronger drugs particularly heroin by the time I was eighteen and spent a year or so abusing that substance but managed, mostly by lucky circumstance to quit using it, although I would come back to it many times over the next couple of decades until it, along with anything else I could lay my hands on led to a final rock bottom.

Up to the age of 48, I was to use heroin intermittently and was for all that time a daily user of other drugs. Although I was aware my use of drugs was causing problems in my life, I somehow felt that I was in control as the outside stuff, kids, marriage and my career were still somewhat manageable. My addiction progressed and conversely so did the deterioration of my mental health and my ability to cope with life. I suffered many dark times during the years before I came into recovery, dis-honesty, the inability to really look at myself and denial around my dependence issues were causing untold damage in my life for myself and those around me. During these years, I had also become increasingly aware of my sexuality being opposite to the way I lived my life. No matter how I tried to suppress this unwelcome truth the realisation that I was gay began to haunt me, I literally didn't have the tools to deal with it, I also genuinely loved my wife and my family but was living a lie. Denial, avoidance and using drugs to numb me were becoming less effective and the pain it brought was at times unbearable.

The increasing drug use I needed to cover up the toxic effect of secrecy began to take its toll. Year after year as this illness progressed so too did the confusion and turmoil in me, it created anger and resentment, and although I loved my wife and family my inability to handle life and the increasing difficulties my addiction brought left me in a kind of paralysed hopelessness.

Decline

Eventually, my marriage fell apart, primarily down to my drug use. The next seven years were a daily battle to keep some order in my life, for the children, and for work but inevitably my drug habit won out and everything just crashed around me. At the end of my use or rock bottom, I was hollowed out as a person, totally broken. I had managed to get off Methadone but was still abusing pain medications and huge quantities of alcohol. I was living with my father who didn't really want me there, and we had just lost my mother from this disease. I was truly messed up, and suicidal, but somehow, I finally admitted defeat and reached out for help.

I found a place in rehab. After a few weeks in treatment this time (I had gone there a year prior to this and walked out), I had some sort of breakthrough, found some hope and courage and began to think that it might be possible for me to live a life without drugs. I found the humility I needed to accept I was powerless over drugs and really embraced the help offered there. I came into recovery for the first time and began to understand that my issues had less to do with the substance and more to do with my mind. Getting well took a couple of false starts but I settled and began to address some of the issues that had me trapped in my mind. One such issue was my inability to accept or embrace my sexuality, and when (with help) I finally 'came out' in a recovery program I was attending I began to heal somewhat. Nonetheless, I needed real help to start changing a life-time of self-abuse, and to take small actions to bolster my mental health, change my attitude of negativity and find my feet in a fellowship. I remained substance-free for the next five or six years and everything in my life began to improve including my relationship with my family. I was blessed in that sense. Those initial few years were really happy times for me, and the work to look after my recovery seemed to repay me in spades.

Recovery

Recovery for me is always moving and changing as my awareness and experience grows and this process continues the more I interact with other recovering addicts, work with a sponsor, and practice a way of living designed to keep my mental health in good order. I am now two years back in recovery, an achievement I have only managed with the help of others and trying as best I can to live one manageable day at a time. I am often grateful for this wisdom, as keeping myself well, with help, for just one day seems possible. I follow a set of 'guidelines' that are pretty much the opposite of how I lived in active addiction. When I am using the whole axis of my life becomes the substance, be it alcohol or heroin or whatever, the substance itself is not so important, but everything in my life will turn on this axis and become the driving force behind how I operate in the world. When I am taking drugs the most important thing becomes taking drugs and the more I take, the more I crave, despite my life immediately becoming toxic. I begin to distance myself from the things that are good in my life. I become centred on myself, dis-honest, and sink into a state of mind which is not rational, constant use of something which brings me chaos and destruction is hardly sane. A hugely important fact that I need to keep in mind is that even without actively taking a mind-altering substance my thinking can become toxic very quickly if I neglect to care for and maintain a state of recovery, this is where my mental health and my addiction cross borders. If I let myself become complacent, I begin to forget I have a disorder with the power to distort and disturb my thinking, I will revert to that place of insanity. I speak here from experience. I have tools in recovery to watch my thinking, this requires self-assessment, acceptance that this needs to be done constantly and most importantly being around like-minded people. Only then as a part of something bigger can I gain the distance I need to see things as they really are. In my first period of recovery, I had to make drastic changes to my mindset, using the knowledge I had learned about this condition and about myself, I had to become open about the pain of the shame and guilt I carried, look at the past honestly and set about amending some of the wrongs I had brought to the people around me. As a result of this work, I remained in a good state of mind and was capable of looking outward to consider others and care for them. I was blessed during this period to have been able to care for my Dad, whose struggle with dementia had reached a stage where he needed twenty-four help, I managed to keep him in his home until the end. After the death of my father, I launched myself back into life, re-training for another career, I was in a relatively new relationship, and I moved home to a peaceful part of the country. The one thing I didn't do was re-establish my connection to my network of support which had diminished during the time caring for my father, this was a grave mistake as I slowly but surely isolated myself from the very practices that kept me well. Eventually, the rigours of life, the stresses that work brought and another relationship ending badly I was back in emotional pain and had placed myself almost unknowingly apart from the very things that had given me a better life in the first place. When I began to struggle internally in this state of mind, an emotional and mental relapse at first until I reached for the one crutch I had historically used to soothe me, I was immediately and effectively back into active addiction. This last relapse was, in fact, a series of using episodes with gradually diminishing periods of clean time in between. Once released again by taking that first hit, my disease becomes stronger than my resolve however franticly I scrabbled to get back to a place of sanity and order. Towards the end of this battle, I was utterly devastated, physically I was in bad shape and mentally I was back in a state of turmoil and losing hope by the day. Thankfully with my children's support, love and compassionate help, I landed back in a rehab centre door to door from a hospital bed. I would not have made it alone, this I am sure of, I am only here to write this because of my children fighting for me. More than ever now I understand that the work, actions and faith in my ability to recover alongside my peers in recovery take top priority, as alone I cannot fight something which is more powerful than me.

Mental Health

I am, in general, content, and positive when in recovery, there is much in my life to be grateful for and I am a great believer in the incredible benefits I reap when I take any small action to care for myself. By taking my state of being, mental, physical and spiritual into consideration and taking some positive action towards wellness I am already better disposed to seeking solutions rather than becoming paralysed by fear or depression. Nonetheless, I still get days when I can be depressed, or anxious or feel overwhelmed and it is in these episodes that I need to have some self-compassion, to try to accept that I am recovering from a lifetime of self-abuse. This takes time and giving myself the space to feel feelings stemming from present difficulties or the past, and to accept where I'm at in any one day (and that feelings won't kill me) is usually my first action to take. I find the less likely I am to cover up or deny to myself or others the reality of feeling depressed, the more I have control over how I feel. This action of honesty is important for me because it goes against my default position of deluding myself that I can fix myself by myself, self-deception and not taking ownership of how I feel has been, and can still be, the first step in the wrong direction. The 'we' element of peer support and my belief in the power of that alongside a sense of spiritual goodwill available to me, help to achieve a state of mind where delusional thinking, denial, pride and a warped sense of reality don't hold sway over me.

Having peer support and professional therapy has been a huge advantage for me in my recovery journey. Without the help and guidance of others, I wouldn't be where I am today. My support system can help me recognise when my behaviour is lacking, when I'm not reacting appropriately to situations, and when I'm too self-absorbed to see what's happening around me.

Overall, truthfully sharing my experience with others has been crucial in my ability to grow and change as a person. The support and guidance of others have been invaluable in my recovery journey, and I'm grateful to those who have had the courage to hold me accountable and help me recognise areas in which I need to improve.

While I fully believe in the benefits that bonding and sharing with like-minded people brings, and the benefits of therapy I in no way want to exclude or underestimate the power of a loving family in keeping me well and recovering. I am one of the very fortunate people who suffer from addiction problems to still have a family who loves me, supports me and provides that belonging that I crave as a human but yet turn away from when my head is not right. Somehow my family have been able to see past the sickness and see me. For this chance to heal together is, for me, like asking for the impossible and nonetheless receiving it unconditionally. Recovery for a person who has used and abused substances, people, and himself can be hard sometimes but the rewards are nothing short of incredible. As I recover, so too do my family and loved ones around me. Another powerful tool of recovery for me is, through attending meetings etc. I come to witness positive changes in fellow addicts that demonstrate to my cynical mind that it is possible to change one's mindset and attitudes, to change the way we perceive things, to how we react and respond to life and to lead a more contented existence. I see this in the people I prefer to surround myself with now and their example fills me with hope and gives me the courage to work towards positive change within me.

Change

In the process of change and taking responsibility for my life and gaining further insight into how my mind works and has worked in the past, I find the affirmative action that setting pen to paper in twelve-step work with the guidance of a fellow addict sharing his own experience with me, is invaluable in helping me to see things clearly, discarding those traits and behaviours that cause problems for me and addressing my role in harms to others is invaluable. I have learned that some of my thinking and the behaviours that follow are detrimental to me, my mental health and above all to the people around me. Addiction is regularly referred to as 'a family disease' in recovery therapy circles and there is surely evidence of this in my life. I have undoubtedly brought much pain to those whom paradoxedly I love the most. In order to address the hurts I have caused in my addiction I need to understand that there is no real value in an apology without the commitment to do the utmost to not repeat the same hurt. I do my best in this endeavour daily. Gaining some insight and awareness is useless to me unless I take steps to change the attitudes and behaviours that no longer serve me well and build a toolset of new values, work to develop a more productive and positive outlook on life and strive for some kind of humility. With the help of others, I have been given a choice; wallow in the misery remorse and regret can bring or set about making peace with the past and doing my utmost to set things right as far as possible, especially with my family and friends. It is in the realm of relationships, including my relationship with myself that my drive towards self-destruction has caused the most damage, so therefore it is this sphere where I need to concentrate my efforts.

To begin to recover I had to become honest, with others and most of all with myself. It's about growing up, taking responsibility, taking ownership of my choices and decisions going forward and being accountable for the consequences of those choices. To fully face myself, I have had to work with my past, not ignore it nor deny it but use it to understand what has driven me, what mistakes I've made, most times repeatedly and make an internal commitment to look, learn and hopefully create a better future for myself. To recover from addiction, at its core a self-absorbed state of mind, I find now that when I look outward, when I can be useful or helpful in the lives of others, I become a more contented person at heart, this is one of the joys of being substance-free and having a clear mind. Recovery takes work, there is no doubt about it and it's not for the faint-hearted, but it is possible to recover one day at a time and there are many hundreds of thousands of recovering addicts worldwide to attest to that, so this is what I try to remember when I falter. There is at the beginning, an element of blind faith required in reaching for it, especially when one is so disillusioned and disempowered it can seem impossible, I am glad to be part of a collective effort to dispel that doubt and bring some hope to other addicts who, like me cannot recover alone.

I have lost my Mother and two of my closest friends to this, so often a fatal disease and not a month goes by when I don't hear of another person losing their life in some way related to addiction, often a person I have known. I am right now, right here, so incredibly grateful for this gift of recovery, another chance to grab life and a chance to heal. My addiction is just a part of me, like my sexuality and my work and being a dad, a friend, and a brother, it will always be a part of me but it does not have to define me, like all parts of me it makes me who I am as a person, and I am proud these days to say my name is Paul. So no one part defines me but rather all of these aspects make me who I am today. I try to make amends for the past as I move forward, and I do my best each day to protect and cherish this chance to live and recover one step at a time. I am a fortunate man indeed.

Chapter 14

Arlene's Pathway to Recovery

Arlene

My Childhood

I am the youngest of three children and grew up in a small bungalow in a little village, with our parents. My dad was disabled from a young age and due to the nature of his disability he was unable to work outside of the home. My mother would go out two evenings a week to work in the local pub. This meant that my parents were always struggling financially. However, we always had what we needed, not necessarily everything we wanted, but definitely everything we needed.

My parents' marriage was a happy one and I only ever remember them having one argument during the course of my childhood.

As my sister got old enough to 'supervise' my brother and I, on a Sunday night – and only on a Sunday night – my dad would head down to the pub while Mam worked and have 2 or 3 pints of Guinness and they would come home together. My parents were not big drinkers and I rarely ever witnessed them even merry.

Teenage Years

When I started secondary school, I was only 11. I had wanted to go to a mixed school where my brother attended but my dad would not agree and sent me to the all-girls school that my older sister attended. She loved it there, but as alike as we are in some ways, we are like chalk and cheese in others. From the get go I hated school. I made great friends and had great fun with them but the school side of things did not appeal to me at all. I effortlessly achieved really good grades, so there was no stress that way but I just did not like it.

I remember one time my English teacher, a lovely kind elderly lady, asked me to stay after class. She was concerned about me as she noticed I was distracted and I hadn't turned in an essay on time. It was me she was concerned about, not the essay. I ended up breaking down in tears and telling her that my dad was having an affair and that things at home were not good. Bless her, she even changed my

Different Diagnoses, Similar Experiences:
Narratives of Mental Health, Addiction Recovery and Dual Diagnosis, 117–121
Copyright © 2024 by Arlene
Published under exclusive licence by Emerald Publishing Limited
doi:10.1108/978-1-80455-848-520241014

grade on my report to make my life that bit easier. At this stage, I was about 14. I began to feel real anger towards my dad for what he was doing. He would bring this woman to our house and for some reason my mother, although obviously deeply hurt, put up with it. Naturally, he pretended nothing was going on but I knew. We all did. He's a terrible liar.

When it came to transition year and getting work experience, I had no idea what I wanted to do so I decided to go working with my Mam in the pub. The first night I collected glasses and by the second night, I was pulling pints. I took to it like a duck to water and loved working with my mother. I was always Daddy's girl but this had changed and I was finally getting to know my mother as a person, and it was beautiful. I spent 7 years working weekends in the pub with her.

My first drink was when I was 16 and it was Baileys. I liked the taste but it was only ever the odd one I would have some nights after work while my mam would have her pint, before we'd clean up and go home.

I started dating a boy when I was 17 and this was when I started to go out to drink socially. We might go out once every 5 or 6 weeks and I would drink 4 or 5 bottles of alcopops. I would sometimes be tipsy but never drunk. I would remember everything. The worst thing that ever happened was that I might get emotional over my dad, who had moved out when I was 16.

The Beginning of the End

At the age of 22, I bought my own home. Impressive, people say, but it was also a massive responsibility and I worked very hard for it.

Roughly two years later I met John, the man I was to spend the next 14 years with. The father of my two beautiful sons. He was incredibly handsome, kind, considerate and loving... for about a year. Gradually, bit by bit all that disappeared, and I became trapped in hell. The reality is that John was a controller, a manipulator, a narcissist, a bully and a misogynist. He cheated, he lied and for want of a better word, he 'mind-fucked'.

I changed every part of my being trying to please him but now, being more educated on the matter, know that I never could.

He would call me 'uneducated, unemployable and unattractive'. Bare in mind that he would not allow me to work so I stayed at home to mind our boys. I spent all my time with the kids and he was always absent. I don't regret my time with them and myself and the boys were extremely close.

In 2015, my Mam was diagnosed with stage 4 lung cancer. Devastation doesn't even describe how I felt. How we all felt. My sister, brother and I cared for Mam in her own home around the clock for 19 months until she passed away at the age of just 56.

During the time of her illness, before things got bad, most nights someone would be over to visit and drinks would always be on offer. I was already suffering at home and I would regularly join in on the drinking which at this stage was vodka and coke. I would come home late and go out to the back garden to my Labrador and hug him and cry because there was no one else. My brother and sister were obviously dealing with mam's illness but they had supportive partners they could talk to. For me, it was the dog.

I remember my mother used to comment at times about how fast I used to drink, and the fact that I always held the glass in my hand rather than put it down. At this point, if I did get out for a night, I would have blackouts.

Regaining and Losing Myself Simultaneously

In 2018, a year after losing mam, I decided that I wanted to regain some respect from John and I went back to college. He was not happy.

Things had become so bad between us that I would go to bed as early as was 'acceptable' and sneak a bottle of wine up to bed, to drink before he'd come up, in a bid to be asleep before he would arrive. I was drinking this along with my sleeping tablets. But of course, it was only on occasion I would do this. Like, once or twice a week.

Then COVID-19 hit and John had to work from home. Thankfully I had a part-time job by now, 2 days per week in an 'essential service' but I was also now doing another course, but it was online now. I was on five courses consecutively, some even simultaneously just to escape my relationship. Every single time I was up in the room at my desk I was drinking some form of alcohol. I was a high-functioning alcoholic to say the least. Though I wouldn't admit this to myself. I told myself I had it under control and if I wasn't in the relationship, I was in I wouldn't be doing this. The relationship might have driven me there but at this stage, addiction had well and truly sunk its jaws into me.

In the end, I was working two part-time jobs, doing my courses online two nights per week and drinking most nights. I was class rep most of the time and I achieved first-class honours in every single one of those courses.

John began to cop on. He would call me an alcoholic, even though he had no idea the extent I was drinking. What else would a loving partner do in that situation except buy a bottle of wine and tell me he was putting it in the fridge for me. He wanted me to fail. He wanted me weak. As bad as I may have wanted those bottles of wine he kept buying me, I never touched one. Of course, I would supply myself privately.

In 2020, I attended a family funeral and naturally, went back to the pub with the family for drinks. As it was my father's side of the family which I didn't see very often, I was enjoying the catch and the drinks were flowing. One of my uncles kept handing me glasses of wine. I don't even know how many I had but these days I was not able to handle it. We had gone to the pub at 3 p.m. and at 6 p.m. I woke up with a bloody nose, a black eye and torn clothing after being raped at the hands of my father's brother.

I was brought to the hospital and the house was sealed off for forensics. All the proper exams were done on me in the correct time frame. The guilt I felt was massive even though the sergeant that accompanied me for the exam in the sexual assault treatment unit assured me again and again that my being drunk didn't make a difference. It wasn't my fault. But it felt like my fault.

Despite immense pressure and threats from John to press charges, I couldn't. I simply could not deal with the unnatural on goings of my relationship, protect my children and deal with a trial.

In 2021, my relationship ended the hard way, with a barring order to get him out of the house. For this, I would pay.

The children adjusted quite quickly but I was really conflicted because I still loved this man but I couldn't live the way I had and things had been getting dangerous for the children as the abuse was intensifying. I missed the boys terribly the days and nights they were at their dad's and as the relationship had alienated me from most people, I would spend most days and nights drinking and sleeping. One day, while the boys were at school, I took a sleeping tablet and went to bed. When I got up, I thought I was fine and poured myself a glass of wine to have before they got home. When the boys came in from school, they knew I was not 'right' and they rang their dad. Their dad rang the guards, and the guards placed the boys in his care that day. The very next day I received a letter from his solicitor notifying me that he was applying for sole custody. Bingo. Just what he was waiting for. The court awarded him the custody and I lost them. I had to fight hard for any access. One glass of wine and a sleeping tablet and my life changed forever. Of course, I know I had a problem, now, but on that day, it was one glass of wine.

Fight for My Life

After my sister begged me to go into residential treatment for weeks and I flat out told her to stop bringing it up because it was not happening, I eventually had a serious chat with myself and a look at my life. I needed help and could not do it on my own, clearly. I decided I did want residential treatment after all, and once I made this decision I couldn't get there fast enough. I had my assessment in Aiseiri in Cahir with the legendary J.T. on Thursday and he offered me a bed for the next day. I was actually excited!

I embraced the programme and got on with the start of my recovery. My first night in Aiseiri was the first night in over 10 years that I slept like a baby. I was safe. No crazy men, no alcohol, no phone. Just peace, structure and probably most importantly – no shame. By the time I left Aiseiri, I was nearly sad to leave but excited about the new me, whoever that might turn out to be. I felt like I'd never even want a drink again. I was attending AA and SMART recovery meetings and meeting new people in recovery. And most importantly I was attending my aftercare meetings with Aiseiri.

Then 3 months later I was hammered and driving up the road to drink on the roadside and driving back. Lunacy! 'Why did I drink?' you ask? The sky is blue. The grass is green. The dog barked. Take your pick. The answer is that I do not know. I am an alcoholic. I am definitely an alcoholic. That is something I do well to remember. Aiseiri moved me into a relapse group and I remain sober, for today.

My recovery has given me a voice again and I am in the process of a custody battle. This time the courts are listening to me. There is only one thing now that can stand in the way of me having my children back and that is a drink. I can do anything else in the world that I choose. But not drink. That's what I have to keep reminding myself. And it is not easy. I'm constantly battling with myself but although I am in very early recovery, I am already seeing the results. My life is changing. I still don't know who I am fully. I am many, many things. But I am also an alcoholic. If I don't look after myself and keep my recovery as my top priority, then I lose it all again.

While I am in this minefield of recovery, my addiction is on the sidelines doing press-ups, sharpening its claws and waiting to sink its jaws into me again.

I pray, that it doesn't. For today.

Chapter 15

Jack's Hope

Jack Kilkenny

Hi, I'm Jack and I'm an alcoholic and an addict. If you're reading this book, then you are looking for the help I once looked for. I took up drinking and taking drugs at a young age, my addiction escalated to cocaine and prescription drugs. When I was at the end of my active addiction, I was all alone in my bedroom in my Mam's house, snorting lines of cocaine off my bedroom locker and urinating into bottles, because I was too paranoid to even go to the bathroom, which was two doors down from my own bedroom. I got to the stage of active addiction and I had no friends left. I also was left with no car or apartment. No one would talk to me because I was too out of control and I was hanging around with the wrong people, which led me to having run-ins with the law on more than one occasion.

My life is not like that today. I found recovery when I went into residential treatment in Hope House and Fellowship House. These two treatment centres helped me battle my addiction and got me on the road to recovery. I found peace and solace in the rooms of Narcotics Anonymous and Alcoholics Anonymous. I have a sponsor who is bringing me through the steps, and I go to around two or three meetings a week, and my aftercare. I am over eighteen months clean and sober, and this is because I am doing all the right things that were suggested to me. If you are struggling at the moment, trust me, put your hand out and ask for help. You won't regret it, and you'll have a nice clean and sober life!

Different Diagnoses, Similar Experiences:
Narratives of Mental Health, Addiction Recovery and Dual Diagnosis, 123–123
Copyright © 2024 by Jack Kilkenny
Published under exclusive licence by Emerald Publishing Limited
doi:10.1108/978-1-80455-848-520241015

Chapter 16

My Story

John

Recovery College South East, Ireland

As far as I can recollect, my first taste of a mood-altering substance was a bottle of black and white whiskey from my parents' drinks cabinet when I was probably around 13 years old. Nothing exceptional, just a few sips with some friends. I wasn't sure if I liked the taste but I did like the sense of excitement, exploration and the stronger bond with my friends that I got from it. I also liked that it gave me a sense of being an adult.

Prior to this, I did need to be pumped out in the hospital having swallowed a bottle of Junior Disprin which at the time was orange flavoured and tasted like any other sweets from the shop. That was when I was 3 years old so it was probably more to do with innocence and misplaced medication than a desire to get high.

It was when I was 13/14 that I was first introduced to cannabis. I was hanging around with an older group and starting to get into the music scene. We would drink cider, smoke cannabis and use inhalants like glue and lighter fuel to get high. It was all very easy, fun and for me it gave me a real sense of belonging, being a part of something and having a positive identity.

This behaviour was largely limited to summertime as I was in secondary school by now, although, any holidays from school meant I reverted back to this way of life. Christmas in particular was spent in the pub as much as possible for a 14-year-old.

By the time I was in 3rd year, I was smoking cannabis more regularly and drinking at weekends. However, this time coincided with the older group I was with leaving for London for work. Ireland, in the early 1980s, was a time of high unemployment and for many London was the answer.

When this happened, I fell into another peer group, the drugs stopped but the drinking kept up. My fashion sense changed and I turned from punk to trendy. The pubs I went to changed also. I was happy at this time, chasing girls, getting into relationships and living for the weekend. Life seemed pretty normal and

Different Diagnoses, Similar Experiences:
Narratives of Mental Health, Addiction Recovery and Dual Diagnosis, 125–128
Copyright © 2024 by John
Published under exclusive licence by Emerald Publishing Limited
doi:10.1108/978-1-80455-848-520241016

enjoyable. I had returned to my love of boxing as well as joining a local gym to lift weights. In hindsight, the 5th and 6th years of secondary school were two very happy years in my life.

In 1990, I finished my leaving cert and with it, school was a thing of the past. It coincided with the return to Ireland of many who had emigrated to London in the early 1980s. Ireland was opening up and many social changes were beginning to happen. Employment was increasing and things seemed positive.

This was a critical time in my life. I often think school was the scaffolding that was keeping me together because when it finished my life fell apart in some ways. This was the first time I felt really depressed. I remember being out drinking with some friends who had returned from London and at the end of the night I was suicidal, wanting to end my life and crying like a child. It was a weird experience for me and one which I quickly buried beneath a hardened outer image, shame and simply ignoring what had happened. It was never spoken of again, especially to the friend with whom I had broke down in front of.

I need not be surprised as I had challenges with my moods, thoughts and emotions throughout my life. I was a sensitive child who was deeply affected by mental health challenges in my family, alcoholism amongst older siblings and occasional domestic violence. It made me live in fear and always guess when the next argument or drama would unfold. I believe this was the reason that I sought belonging outside of my family unit and sought acceptance from my peers through risk-taking behaviour.

From 1990 to 1994 my drug use was everyday but limited to alcohol and cannabis. I worked throughout my addiction which probably kept me somewhat grounded. With the return of more and more people from London and the onset of the rave scene, my drug use was to change dramatically. Ecstasy and amphetamine were introduced to me and I fell completely in love with these types of drugs. The effect they had on me was so positive that I just kept chasing that hit all over again and again. Where cannabis had made me feel inward, quiet and even paranoid, ecstasy and amphetamine gave me all the confidence I never had, they made me feel positive, sociable and outward. I felt I had found what I was missing in life.

The next drug I used was cocaine. This really brought me to a very dark place. At first, the drug gave me a lot of confidence, self-belief and a general good feeling about life. It provided me with something to live for and in hindsight, it was at times my whole world. The getting, using and giving up of cocaine was a very powerful sequence or pattern over a number of years.

It was during my addiction to cocaine that I really lost myself and felt most disconnected from myself and the world around me. Contact with family members was minimal, I lived in a different area of the country and so it was easy to isolate, disconnect and hide my addiction. My love for exercise, sport and socialising was completely destroyed and I lived a very unhealthy lifestyle. There were periods where I would have binged on alcohol and cocaine for days on end without any food, sleep or contact with other people except for those who were using with me. Much of this time though was spent alone, on reflection, my addiction was a descent into loneliness, isolation, self-loathing and self-destruction.

The last year of my using was characterised by a deep sense of hatred of myself and a desire to harm myself. I remember using cocaine in an effort to hurt myself and could not get enough of it to satisfy this desire such was my unease and rejection of myself.

Perhaps a saving grace initially for me was that I always maintained a good work ethic and in between binges over the years I always held down work and had a loving partner who was there to welcome me back to the real world after my binges. This however, could not last, obviously there are limits to employers and partners tolerance levels and rightly so. The fact though that I never completely let go of life tells me that deep down my spirit was strong and something helped me hold on. After all, I loved life at the same time as hating it – a paradox of addiction perhaps – and one which when I look back I often wonder what it was all about.

I was introduced to recovery in 2002 by a work colleague who spotted something in me that he himself was living with. That being addiction, in his case, alcoholism. He had found recovery through Alcoholics Anonymous and could see the despair in my whole being while coming back from a binge or just the general depression that I was carrying and thought I was hiding so well.

I went along to my first AA meeting with him and found the experience a bit uncomfortable in that it was a small and intimate setting, people were talking honestly about their life, their recovery and the problems they had overcome due to following the 12-step programme.

I also found out about Narcotics Anonymous which I started to attend but just could not commit to it. I attended a drug addiction counsellor also. A lot of my motivation was being driven by fear. Fear of the mess my life was, fear of owing money for drug debts and fear of my partner finally having enough of me. It was a horrible time in my life and eventually, I crashed. My partner left and I fully understand now why she did but at the time I was so self-consumed that I found that hard to deal with. I was desperate and so I rang an addiction treatment centre near my home town and got on to a waiting list. This meant sick leave from work and when a place became available I went in for four weeks of treatment which involved one-to-one therapy, group therapy and 12-step work.

Life was great upon completion of this treatment but it did not last long. I had many issues and challenges ahead and it was all too easy to revert back to using drugs as a means of escaping the reality of my situation. The drug debts were still there, the relationship issues, the sadness, the numbness and strained relations with family members were all very difficult. On top of this, the psychological pull of cocaine was immense and in 2003 the economy was booming, there were lots of drugs around. In 2004, I relapsed having been off drugs for 6 months. It was devastating and the following two years were of a similar nature where I would get clean and then go back to using.

Peer support kept me going though and I had made a few close friendships in NA that were always reliable and willing to offer support when I asked for it. While I was struggling in those moments, the bigger picture was that I was heading in the right direction and eventually in 2006 I entered a very progressive and person-centred residential house for people struggling in their recovery. I don't tend to use words dramatically but this experience was life-changing and I have no hesitancy in saying that it saved my life.

In particular, it was the manager of the house that was the catalyst for change for me. His way was kindness, acceptance and non-judgmental in everything he did and every way he met people. In my time here, I enrolled for third-level education, I was introduced to meditation, compassion, and really found my love of life again. I found support through others in a similar journey in life, I was able to be of support also and I got a good grounding in recovery.

I was listening to speaker tapes of Eckhart Tolle, Anthony Mellow and Joseph Campbell who in particular had a profound impact on my thinking, my attitude and released my curiosity to a level where I just seemed to excel in finding and maintaining recovery and a new way of life.

I left this treatment centre in 2007, I had lived there for over a year and I have not looked back in terms of drug use. I have gone on to achieve several third-level qualifications, I have a good job and career now that I enjoy and I have quality relationships around me including a beautiful young son.

Recovery has given me a certain sense of security that I know I am there for my son and my family and I like to acknowledge the help and support I received to get me where I am. That is why I see recovery as being possible for everyone, no one is a lost cause and miracles do happen. I have seen recovery happen for people who have been written off by society and by themselves.

In recent years, I have been introduced to other recovery thoughts. When the drugs stopped for me, over time, my mental health became more apparent to me. Anxiety, depression, stress, paranoia and an overthinking mind all contribute to impacting life in a challenging way. At times, they prevent me from doing things I want to do. Recovery has allowed me to explore my life through therapy, counselling, and confronting trauma and its impact. I have built a whole array of coping skills and ways to manage in life.

The question of cause and effect in terms of addiction and mental health arises often. These days I accept I will never fully answer this question but my experience tells me that my life was shaped by events that would have made me prone to anxiety, worry and fear. In addition, drugs perhaps offered an escape from this, self-medicating in some ways. Maybe chronic use of hard drugs had an effect on my mental health also and so the cause and effect may be a two-way process.

While NA and other resources listed above have built me back up as a person, it is the CHIME framework in mental health recovery that has brought my recovery forward to a more complete transformation. When I look back, it is the elements of connection, hope, identity, meaning and empowerment that were at play all along. CHIME for me is an easy reference to check myself against as I strive to live the best life I can and to live my life to the fullest.

Chapter 17

We're So Much Stronger than We Think

Mark Coyle

I grew up with four brothers and one sister and my dad drank a lot when we were younger and I hated it. With this hatred of seeing my father drunk all the time, I thought I would be immune to this, well I was SO WRONG. My problems with alcohol started in my 20s. I was drinking for fun and this was my reward. Then over the years, I drank more to cope with the stresses of life, I was a functional alcoholic that lived day by day with alcohol as my medicine to keep me going. Little did I know that alcohol was a depressant itself and this was where the anxiety bounced into my life and this made it harder for me to perform daily tasks in life.

It was shortly after my wedding I stopped drinking in 2017. After returning from my honeymoon and working six days a week, I felt panic attacks coming on and also I was not feeling the best physically (I could not stand up) and mentally (panic attacks) so I went to the Emergency Department. I was kept in hospital for over three weeks and was given diagnosis of acute pancreatitis due to drinking heavily over the years. I spent time in the hospital in high dependence; I was in blackness for three weeks, not only in detox but also hearing voices and having terrible dreams I even pulled out a feeding tube at one stage. I swore I'd never be in this place again for this so I started my recovery journey with the help and support of a social worker who introduced me to recovery. After all the physical and mental pain and detox in which I have endured within these three weeks in the hospital has been one of the most frightening experiences in my life. I began my recovery journey in August 2017 after being released from the hospital on lifetime medication for acute pancreatitis.

As starting off in my recovery journey I couldn't function as I needed a drink so I was introduced to a Treatment Centre in Ballymun. During my treatment, I learned a lot about myself in which includes my new surroundings which were my family, whom now were all strangers to the sober Mark. The downside I became like my dad moaning about all the things I used to let slide, I became insurable to my family (consisting of two stepchildren my wife and my daughter). I had anger and unsolved problems and my availability to overlook things was gone, there was a big change in me. I started to resent my family as I was fresh in recovery,

Different Diagnoses, Similar Experiences:
Narratives of Mental Health, Addiction Recovery and Dual Diagnosis, 129–131
Copyright © 2024 by Mark Coyle
Published under exclusive licence by Emerald Publishing Limited
doi:10.1108/978-1-80455-848-520241017

I became alone in my own recovery and I had no one to share and understand this experience I was going through except one freaking hour a week in this treatment centre for addiction.

After being on a waiting list for counselling eventually I went to counselling once a week to discuss what was bothering me and learned different techniques to relieve stress in my recovery. Having a therapist who believed me that I could do well in recovery and reach my goals over time; this has helped so much in my confidence. With my confidence coming back slowly, I took up jogging that I never thought I'd be fit to do. Surprisingly I loved jogging and this was a way to have control of my life again in a positive and healthy habit and hopefully leave bad habits (alcohol) behind. I was attending support groups and met other like-minded people that had been through similar journeys that I have been through and this was so empowering knowing I was not alone. I was eating well, broccoli for breakfast and before I knew it over time I was running 10k marathons and feeling life again all while losing my family along the way.

After two years, my marriage split up and this was a sad occasion for my wife, my stepchildren and my daughter. I was heartbroken and I had a sense of abandonment and this made my recovery more difficult as I moved back to my parents' home in which I left six years earlier with a sense of relief and to return once again was not good. This was the biggest step I have taken in my entire life (never mind sober) as I moved into my parents' house I felt triggers and lots of memories coming back to me as a child, some were good and a lot not so good. Then COVID-19 came and my job shut down, I was sofa surfing in my parents' house with no address or no job and most importantly I had NO IDENTITY. I was lost and my moral compass was shattered. This was the hardest time for me, I was on the outside looking in at all my drunken adventures and COVID-19 made it worse to believe in recovery during that time however I still had hope. The world was shut down and the strangest thing is the world was like me, however, I was living this life before it became fashionable.

Throughout COVID-19, I had been concentrating on Eva and enjoying spending time with her and we were making the best times, come reality we have a love bond like no other. Lockdown came and went and my job slowly picked up and in the words of Pink Floyd I became comfortably numb. I'm six years sober today while writing this and I wouldn't change a single thing if I ever had the chance again. I have learned that recovery comes with personal responsibility and reaching out and trying different supports such as peer support groups and engaging in recovery led initiatives such as now writing my narrative. Thank you for asking me to write this narrative which gives me more confidence to continue on my recovery journey without feeling guilty or ashamed.

My daughter was the greatest thing to come out of all this and I took up another sort of stepchild along the way. Eva we're not where we want to be but we're so far from what we were, I breath you Ava everyday day in everything I do. Eva, you give me the power to accept the things I cannot change. For that, your life will be plane sailing as I will be blown gently on those sails. I'd like to also thank Eoin, Alex and Belinda and especially my mum who pulled me threw the hard times. I have hope now and a life worth living and that is how recovery has been for me.

After all, we are all stories in the end, let's make it a good one. I leave you this quote by Nathaniel Branden '*The First step towards change is awareness and the second step is acceptance*'.[1]

[1]Goodreads 2024, https://www.goodreads.com/quotes/1356118-the-first-step-towards-change-is-awareness-the-second-step

Chapter 18

Journey to Recovery

Shay

Childhood Years

I was a lonely child until the age of 13 and to say lonely pretty much sums up a lot of my early years. At the age of about 6, we moved to just outside the city and moved to a number of houses while the house was being built. For most of these years, everything from a family perspective was pretty much in good shape and relatively normal. My parents both worked, with my dad working shift hours which had many 'perks' to the job and mam worked in retail. He was the dominant figure in the household.

From 8 or 9 after moving out to the country into a larger house I started to take notice more of what was going on around me. My parents were arguing and this was becoming more frequent. I remember waking up to shouting things crashing and doors banging. I remember lying in darkness in my bedroom and hearing this going on and waiting for the next loud bang to startle me or the door to burst open. Mam followed by dad shouting. This was becoming more frequent and more physical over the next couple of years. Being a lonely child and not having any support or someone to comfort me was having a severe impact on my mental state of mind and confidence. Each night going home I would sit and wonder if this was going to happen again night after night. Having only started drinking later in life in his mid-20s, my father was a really fit man with All Ireland Champion.

One night my mam came into my bedroom after an argument with my dad who had just left the house to the pub. This was to ensure we were gone before he returned home for the second round. My parents separated when I was around 10 for the first time and my mam and I spent Christmas in her home place with relatives. This would now be our home for about 2 years until they reunited. I did not talk about what was going on in our home nor did I have anyone to talk to about what I was going through as a child and didn't realise what impact this was having on me.

Different Diagnoses, Similar Experiences:
Narratives of Mental Health, Addiction Recovery and Dual Diagnosis, 133–138
Copyright © 2024 by Shay
Published under exclusive licence by Emerald Publishing Limited
doi:10.1108/978-1-80455-848-520241018

Round 2

After getting back together again things seemed good for a while until my dad's drinking started getting heavier and the fighting started again. He was a very dominant figure in the house and you felt like you were walking on eggshells all the time around him. Although he wasn't physical with me, when fighting with my mam things were getting more physical and at the age of 11 this was having a pretty significant impact on how I was perceiving the world and having this fear in my home. My mam then fell pregnant and me being a lonely child took this rather hard initially as my whole life was about to change. Was this reaction down to the fact I would now be sharing the home with another sibling and not getting everything, I wanted? No, this was more down to introducing a vulnerable baby into a home that was becoming more and more chaotic and violent and fearing for my mother.

1 + 1 = 2

My sister was born when I was 12 and this was an excellent time in my life as there was this new life in our home and I was the big brother there to support and protect her. Everything was fine for about 2 years until there were more arguments starting to creep in again and this was happening more frequently. Mam had made the decision one night after dad had left to take the two of us out of the home and move into our own place back in town. At this age, I was hitting my teenage years and life was becoming more difficult and I was going through a rollercoaster of emotions.

Best of Both Worlds

A choice was put to me to choose between spending time with my dad on the weekends and my mams during the week or just staying with my mam full time. I had chosen to stay with my dad on the weekends while my sister was with my mam. For the next few years, my weekends were spent out in my dad's house where at the start everything was fine because there wasn't much alcohol involved. This then changed to him picking me up and going straight to the pub at five until leaving time. I had spent a lot of time in the local pub and most of the weekends were now filled with him drinking throughout and me spending time alone in the house and hiding my father's drinking from friends. I was not able to have friends over at this stage because they were starting to notice and I was feeling ashamed. During this time most other parents were bringing their kids to sports while I was spending my weekends in the pubs. He would drop me back to my mother's on Monday morning. I had not shared what was going on in dads with my mam as I was fearful that I wouldn't see him.

Teenage Years

In school, I also was quite alone and being a small skinny individual, I was intimidated a lot as I didn't have many friends moving to the town school. I was picked on because of my size and was an easy target because I kept to myself, not having the confidence to stick up for myself.

As I got older into my mid-teens I was changing and my dad's drinking got heavier. I always had this fearful feeling and nervousness in myself. From the age of 15, I had started to consume alcohol with my dad and with some friends. There was always alcohol around the house as this was one of the perks of his job. I would sneak cans out of the house after coming home from the pub with my dad and consume more alcohol with my friends down the lane.

My friends and I had started to experiment with hash and weed also around this time which initially this wasn't an issue and I quite enjoyed it. Ignoring the fact that my sister was now spending the weekend also in dads who was heavily drinking for the weekend. One night my mams in town we had been smoking and I was at home on my own after and started to feel a bit uneasy myself. This overwhelming fear and panic started to set in on me and I couldn't calm myself down because I didn't know what was happening to me.

Panic and Fear

I called my mother in a panicked state after smoking weed, telling her what I had done and that I didn't know what was going on at the time. This was the start of what I was told that I was having panic attacks which I am sure I was having earlier in my life. At this point, that it was 'official' or to label the feelings of fear I was having. I was taken to the doctor and was diagnosed as being depressed and prescribed medication to settle the anxiety and panic attacks. On the weekends I would continue to consume alcohol while on medication which didn't help with the anxiety and one fed the other. During the week I wouldn't drink but, on the weekends, I would make up for it because there were no limitations as my father was inebriated most of the time. Mixing the medication with alcohol did nothing for my mental health at the time as I was still a teenager and still striving to find my place. This led to a lot of arguing and fighting with my dad. For most of the week, I would be highly anxious and not drink but still have panic attacks and on the weekends, I would self-medicate with alcohol to cope with the anxiety.

Passing the Torch

Throughout these years there was a lot of anger and resentment towards my dad and life in general for what had happened when I was a child which led to numerous occasions where we would often fight and sometimes come to blows. Was I taking out my anger or just becoming a man not letting myself be put down any longer. It was at this stage of my life that alcohol was starting to consume my life more and more. Was I becoming more and more like my father? He had lost his father at a very young age and had no father figure in his life and I often wonder would history repeat itself.

There were also feelings of responsibility towards him as I could see what alcohol was doing to him and ignored what it was doing to me or at least I couldn't see it at the time. As I became an adult myself, I felt responsible for him and his wellbeing. I was left alone to deal with his alcoholism with no support from any family members. Was this a weight on my shoulders I should take on as a young man or should I have taken a step back to look after myself?

I was angry that he was drinking all the time and through my early twenties, I took on the role of caring for him. I couldn't just walk away and leave him to fade away into the bottom of every bottle.

Young Man

For years I had been on anti-depressants and been to counselling to deal with whatever was going on in my life but quit counselling as I had not felt that it was getting anywhere at the time and felt the medication had done its job. The panic attacks had subdued and my mental health, I felt was in a relatively good place at the time. I was still consuming a lot of alcohol even most of the time during the week but still calling out to my dad during the week to see how he was doing. 99% of the time I would call out to see how he was doing and he would be intoxicated but it was getting too late for me to do anything to help. It had completely consumed his life which was a tough pill for me to swallow but I was following in his footsteps.

Make a Break for It

I held myself back all my life because I felt the responsibility of looking after my father but an opportunity had presented itself to me to try to make a break for myself. Going back to college during the recession I attained a visa to Canada and to go for three months between the first and second year. Having recently broken up with a girlfriend at the time this was a chance for me to try to make a better life for myself. I decided to go by myself to Vancouver to try to get away from everything at home at the age of 28. I got a call from my dad the day I was leaving to say look after yourself and have a good time and he had given me a few bob a few days earlier.

I met 2 guys from Galway on the plane who were block layers and were staying in a hotel just up the road from the hostel I was staying in. I met up with other people in the hostel who were doing a bit of travelling at the time. We hit it off and were out on the lash and partying in Vancouver not a care in the world.

To Be or Not to Be?

One week into my new journey I was after getting back to the hostel after partying most of the night when there was banging on the door of the dorm. The staff at the hostel got into the room and told me there was a phone call at the desk for me. My mother was on the phone and asked me if there was anyone around me but there wasn't. My initial feeling was that something was wrong and I got a knot in my stomach and asked her the question. Was it dad?

She said that my father had passed away and was found dead in the house, he had passed a couple of days ago. Here I was for the first time in my life trying to get away from everything and make a new life for myself but it was not meant to be. I boarded the plane and made my way back to Ireland only to meet a friendly face who happened to be an air host on my journey back who had also lost his father. This eased the journey home and I was met in Dublin airport by my younger sister and cousin. My dad was 52 when he died and had cirrhosis of the liver and was practically the same age as his father when he died.

This was a big blow to me and I had hit the bottle quite hard after this and not dealt with the loss well but decided to take the year out and go back to Canada with a buddy to finish out the visa. Only 10 days into my new journey I got a call from a girl I had been seeing when I had got back the first time to say she was pregnant. While dealing with the loss of my dad I had now another major life-changing moment. Canada was obviously not a place I was meant to be in as my cards were dealt. We had agreed that I stay and come back before the birth to try to make the best of what time I had left in Canada.

Life Changing

For the next 8 months, my mental health started to deteriorate but I didn't do anything about it except drink to cope with the life-changing events that had just happened. I would not have been one for taking drugs and not smoke weed because I knew this hadn't agreed with me. Harder drugs were widely available in Vancouver and I had started to dabble as well as drink vast amounts of alcohol. This was the case for most of my time in Canada and was a way of coping and burying my emotions. All these events that had just happened in such a short space of time had triggered my anxiety and I was back having panic attacks again and getting very low in myself.

Fatherhood

I returned back to Ireland a month earlier than expected to try to get my feet back on the ground and develop a relationship with my now wife. Everything was going well and we had our first child but the alcohol consumption still continued. A couple of years later we had another child but my alcoholism was becoming a lot more evident and starting to take its toll on my life and family life. I knew I had a problem but didn't do anything about it. At this stage, I was having panic attacks every morning and my days were filled with anxiety and fear.

Facing the Facts

My mother and sister had intervened as I had been drinking while taking care of the kids one day and I was in the bad state both mentally and physically. I reached out for help after having an attack while minding the kids while drinking. This led me to go back to counselling and facing up to the fact that alcohol was a problem haven taken over my life. It was only through the counselling that I had realised that I had not dealt with all the childhood trauma and that I was really suffering from anxiety. I was using alcohol as a coping mechanism and just burying my feelings for a few hours a night at the end of a bottle.

Early Recovery

Having finally come to terms with the fact that I was an alcoholic, I tried many times to quit and fell off the wagon but after a few attempts and with the supports in place I finally really dedicated myself and committed to recovery. My mental health had gotten so bad that everyday activities were becoming impossible and life in general was becoming unbearable. I was surviving not living. Months of counselling really put into perspective what was happening, what I went through and how my whole perspective of life had changed over the years of consuming alcohol.

I went to the doctor having had many discussions with family and counselling about taking medication for my anxiety. This was something I was hesitant about as my last experience on anti-depressants was not a good one and coming off them at the time, I had bad experiences and had done it without consulting my doctor. It didn't help the fact that years later I realised that the medication I had previously been on was taken off the market due to its addictive properties and side effects.

Choose Life

I started taking a mild form of anti-depressant/anxiety medication and stopped drinking alcohol. Initially, my recovery was hard as I now had a void in my life that had been filled for so long with alcohol right the way back to my teenage years without me even realising it. History had been repeating itself through three generations and it was now time to break the cycle. My father's father died at 56, my dad had died at 52. I needed to make a change in my life so my sons wouldn't be burying their dad at such a young age. I chose life.

Throughout my life and childhood trauma, I had not realised that I had mental health issues and addiction issues and only through the support of my family and supports I have been able to overcome them. I have met some of the best and most courageous people I know in my recovery journey having battled their own demons that I will hold dear to my heart and support in times of need.

Having been in recovery for over two and a half years now, life is really amazing as recovery has given me the confidence to succeed and overcome many of the obstacle's life throws at us. I now have control over my life, have the choice to live and choose every day to live rather than just survive or exist.

For this, I want to thank my family and friends and the support I have in place which I will forever be in debt to.

Part 4

Dual Diagnosis

Chapter 19

Duelling With Dual Diagnosis

Claire Foy

Dual Diagnosis was a concept I did not learn of until I was in my late 30s and had struggled with being human for the entirety of the previous 3+ decades. For me, I did not have a chance at life until I knew there was such a thing as Dual Diagnosis, and I didn't know that either.

For a long time, I just thought I was a messed-up person who would never fit in and be normal. When I finally came to terms with being an addict, I still could not function, so I figured I must be sicker than every other addict or that I had some kind of issue no one realised and I could not be helped. Somehow, I was different to every other addict, and I would never be a content, competent, consistent human being. Then there were days I thought I was just nuts; I was mentally defective, and I would always want to die and again, I would never be a valuable human being. I did not know that you could be an addict and have a mental illness. And in understanding myself I did so in a way that made me feel alone, crazy and an absolute waste of space on the planet. I used substances to ease the feelings that I was bonkers. I used my mental health issues to explain I was worthless to myself and others so I just stayed in bed and wanted to die. Not knowing that Dual Diagnosis was a real thing and that it was normal meant I struggled for many years trying to fix one and not the other. Trying to use all sorts of substances and people, relationships and obsessions to manage my mental health. My mental health became an insurmountable reason for why I had to use. Using just became the easiest way to escape the pain of being conscious and feeling like I couldn't cope in a complicated world where I had to worry about what others thought of me and where I fit in. Unconscious was always my end goal when I used to. No matter what I used to escape myself; alcohol, benzos, Aerosols, people, sex and work, if I did not get to the point of losing a few hours then it wasn't enough. For me not having to think was the place I always yearned for. I needed a break from me. And struggled for years to find it.

Different Diagnoses, Similar Experiences:
Narratives of Mental Health, Addiction Recovery and Dual Diagnosis, 141–148
Copyright © 2024 by Claire Foy
Published under exclusive licence by Emerald Publishing Limited
doi:10.1108/978-1-80455-848-520241019

Beginning

I grew up in a nice house, in a decent place, with the opportunity of an education and at least the potential to have friends. Within that though I had reasons to justify how worthless I was for a long time. I had three siblings, but I was adopted. My family took me in at seven months old and according to them when they did I was covered in sores and rashes. I am told I was a kid who never cried. Later we assumed this was because the orphanage where I had spent several months just did not respond to crying babies, so I must have just given up.

I, (I assume like most people), do not remember my first thought, but I do remember, as far back as I can, feeling different and lonely and permanently scared. If anything, I remember my childhood like an outsider. Like a movie. A kid in the corner, watching other kids and knowing I had to pretend to be normal. Even before I could articulate it, I knew I was not like every other kid. It started with a constant fear and the things I had to do, (compulsively) to manage whatever it was I was afraid of. For the first 13 years of my life that was the fear that my mother might possibly, suddenly, die. To ensure she didn't die, or no other huge catastrophe would occur in my life I developed a pattern I had to follow. Now I understand it as an obsessive-compulsive disorder, but back then all I knew was that there were some things I had to do, that others didn't which would prevent my mother from dying and other constant intrusive catastrophes I would think up. And I knew I couldn't tell anyone. Because I also knew I wasn't like others. I knew this was something only I was afraid of. At least in my home. None of my other siblings cried themselves to sleep or dived out of moving vehicles because they were afraid to leave their mother in case she would die. I knew I wasn't 'normal' from the earliest points in my life, I didn't know why and I also feared what would happen if anyone knew. I think somehow before I even understood it, I put two and two together and knew that the consequences of not being normal might not be good. And I was also really, really scared because I didn't know what was wrong with me either and why I was so afraid, of everything, all the time. I desperately wanted to be loved so I knew I couldn't afford to be different. Somehow, I knew in my little head that being different and difficult might mean I would not be loved. I can't even put words to how uncomfortable I was with myself, how much of a burden I felt I was even from that early stage.

This constant fear, and worry that never left turned into this pattern of behaviour where, I did everything four times. And I didn't just do it. I had to do it! In my mind not doing it meant the death of those I loved or even myself. It crippled me. I didn't get it but I knew I had to do it. So, I walked down the stairs and had to count the steps in batches of four as I walked. 1, 2, 3, 4. 1, 2, 3, 4. 1, 2, 3, 4. We had 12 steps.

I would count my steps up to four as I walked down the street. I would switch lights on and off four times, and if I thought I ever got the count wrong or missed and lost count I would start from 1 all over again. I would get up and open and close my bedroom door four times. It was incessant, intrusive and impossible to stop. When I think of my childhood I just remember the fear and the counting and the loneliness and the anxiety that someone might catch me doing my rituals.

I am pretty sure living in this world where I had to operate in a somewhat clandestine way much of my waking hours fed into the pre-existing and later consuming paranoia of standing out and being judged

My parents were good parents, but ill-equipped to manage the kid they got, and I am not sure there is a couple out there who could have been equipped for what I brought with me. Outside of that, they had their own stuff too. My dad was a Manic Depressive (now we use the term, Bi-polar). He also had addiction issues in the form of a gambling habit. Daddy, as it happens, too was struggling through Dual Diagnosis but I did not understand that until it was too late for him, and I thought at the time too late for me also. We weren't a dysfunctional family, we functioned. We just functioned badly and how badly depended a lot on how Dad and later how I was doing. I always felt a connection to my Dad. Because somehow, I knew I was as much of a mess as he was. And when things went wrong and we got the blame for everyone else's unhappiness I knew it wasn't fair and I knew neither of us wanted to be how we were or to hurt others or ourselves.

Asking for Help

I saw my first psychiatrist when I was 10. I had continued my obsession with the number four and had woken one day terrified to leave the house and I mean terrified. Again, because my mom might have died while I was out. Now it does not take Freud to figure out what was happening here. Obviously, my being adopted threw me into a loop of catastrophic fear of my mother disappearing which I just couldn't cope with. But it was 1989, and no one in my house had a bogs notion of who Freud was let alone Oedipus, and we could all barely cope with, let alone explain, why I would jump out of moving cars as they tried to get me out of the house, or why I would cry for the entirety of the school day when they did get me in there. Or why I lay awake bawling at night seeking reassurance from my mother, father and anyone else who cared to give it, that they wouldn't die or disappear. It was torture if I am honest, for them and for me and it went on like that for several years. I missed nearly the entirety of fourth class and became the weirdo in the room. Neither students nor teachers had a heap of compassion and I just became the problem kid. I left the house for nothing and no one for the guts of a year and when I did somehow overcome that the constant fear remained and being outside came with severe anxiety that would last for many years later.

Fast forward to 1994, when I was 14. End of the school year. I did what many kids did and decided to steal some alcohol from the house and go to the local park with two friends and try it out. It was a sodding disaster. We got overwhelmingly drunk, at least I did, and they, I assume, felt they had no other choice but to leave me there. But before they did, I decided to kiss one of my (female) friends. And when they did leave, they left me there with a guy we kind of, sort of, knew, who lived in the same area we did. Next thing I remember I am on my back, not really able to move or object, on top of his army jacket. And that is how I lost my virginity. I found alcohol and sex on the same day, and I would never, ever, be the same again. Now I understand what happened to me as rape, but then, I just understood shame and that it was my own fault. I did try to tell someone, but they were adamant it wasn't true, I don't think they could cope if it were, and the only other person I told was too young to help me.

Fast forward again to September that year. I had spent much of that summer in hell. My *'friends'* had decided that kiss made me a lesbian and in their immature wisdom, decided everyone else should know too. So now I was a *'dyke'* and the entirety of my peers both on my street and in my class in school knew. Given it was still a time when being queer was akin to being a leper I was now in a kind of hell I couldn't have even imagined. Now not only did I know I was odd but now everyone else did too.

If I were to tell the entirety of events that led to where I am now, I would need more than a few pages. Suffice it to say by the age of 15, I had found the wrong crowd, was messing around with guys much older than me, using hash, aerosols and ecstasy, having a horrible experience in school and engaging in some serious self-harm and suicidal thoughts while drinking alone in my bedroom. It had gone too far before I even had a chance to figure out where it was going.

Then in desperation, my parents sought help. And it came in the form of an institution I will not name, where I had the privilege of staying for exactly a year, only getting out when they shut the place down. That was not a fun experience, and I spent my time there, learning better techniques to hurt myself from others as naïve, scared, traumatised, alone and confused as I was. While there I got a plethora of diagnoses and by the end of it all feeling just as F**ked up as I was going in. I now had to carry the label of a *'Personality Disorder'* (for me that was and still is a vague title some psychiatrist gives you when in fact they haven't a clue what's going on with you but don't want to admit they haven't got the answer!). When I was released, I had totally forgotten what it was like to live outside that institution and function in a home and the sudden nature of it all left me in a total panic. So, I went back to doing what I knew. I found the same people, drank too much, found other drugs, slept around continued to cut myself and made intermittent attempts to kill myself.

By 18, after a 6-month stint in an adult psychiatric hospital, two miscarriages, torn ligaments, scared arms and a life-threating overdose my family was afraid of me, I was threatening them while under the influence, chasing them with knives and basically performing all kinds of domestic abuse that they felt they had to lock themselves in their bedrooms at night. That's when they kicked me out. They did the right thing and although for many years it hurt me and I blamed them, I know now and have known for a long time not only was it the best thing they could have done but it was the only thing.

Not knowing what to do I spent a week wandering the streets. Then I met an American tourist (someone I still call a friend today) and travelled with him to a destination at the other end of the country and when a couple of weeks later he returned to the US I found an apartment and started a new life. The drug use stopped for a while, and I got a job, in a bar. Then I got another job, in a bar, and then I got another job in a bar. I could not keep a job, mostly because I was a drunk, who only worked in bars. It was a bad life plan. After a few years, I found myself pregnant and alone. And my parents in fear for their grandchild let me come home. Pretty soon I figured out that this meant I could get drunk, get high, and leave my child somewhere safe.

When my parents' marriage finally ran its course, I had no choice but to move out with my daughter as they sold the family home and went their separate ways. By this point, I knew I wanted to be a good mom and I knew I had to do something to increase my chances of being able to support us financially, so I went to college. And I excelled! And they liked me, even respected me. I got awards and I got firsts and I felt for the first time in my life that I was not a complete thick. I had left schools at 15, hadn't taken any formal exams and hadn't opened a book and by the time I was 28, I had a first-class degree and I was starting a PhD with some serious funding.

The three years of my degree were not plain sailing. I had to make a deal with myself not to drink during the academic year bar summer and Christmas. Filling that gap was the obsession with grades and overachieving that in itself would bring me to my knees. On the occasions I did drink, I inevitably also got high if anything was available. I never paid for it. I just slept with the random stranger willing to provide it.

That summer before I started my PhD I decided, right, I'm going to spend the next few years with my head in a book and become a really successful researcher and academic so I'll go nuts and have a hell of a summer. I didn't realise that by the end of the summer, it would be far too late for me to have any control over stopping. I'd started to dip in and out of 12-step programs and read every self-help book from Alan Carr to Oprah Winfrey's recommended list. For the first time, I had gotten to a point where I knew I needed to stop drinking but by then I could not. I was also nursing one of several obsessions I'd had over the years with another guy (he might save my life, you know). It was the weirdest feeling in the world when all I really wanted to do was control how much and how often I drank and I couldn't. At this point, I was a very unfit mother with a child who deserved so much better, but I was hiding it well enough I guess and that is her story and not mine to tell. However, I can't tell this story without sharing what finally broke me. The tipping point came when in a very drunken state I raised my hand and gave my six-year-old a black eye. I could not look at her. I sent her to bed. I spent that night on the stairs with two options. Kill myself or get help. I tried to kill myself many times and failed. And I also swore I would never leave my daughter because I knew how that felt. When my daughter came up to me the next morning and apologised (for the black eye I gave her!), I told her it wasn't her fault, and I was sorry and I would get help now. She had heard it before. She knew I would go to strange meetings to meet strange people, and she knew I saw doctors and psychiatrists, but I had never hit her before and even if she didn't know it, I knew it was my only choice, my last choice, or just give her to my mother. And I couldn't bare the thought of doing that.

By then I had 2 people left in my life. One, a college friend, who for some reason stuck around. Who in my desperation I had told I was a mess and the other a member of a 12-step group I had stopped attending. I rang him, in bits and we talked, and he helped me make the best decision of my life. Then I rang my college friend, and she came straight over with her partner, and they took me to her house, where I stayed for a week before I went into a treatment centre for three months. My mother took my daughter at that time. It was not fun. I lasted the three months, out of guilt and utter desperation. I was as honest as I could be. They made me come off all my meds. And by the end of the first month, I was a bigger mess than I ever had been. I cried more over the loss of alcohol than the pain I had caused or been through.

But treatment didn't cure me, at least not the way I needed it to. I haven't had a drink in nearly 14 years but very quickly after I got out (that 1st night) I started abusing prescription drugs. Something I'd been doing for years. My own prescriptions, sleepers, benzos, and antipsychotics and basically anything I could steal from someone else's meds supply. But hey, I wasn't drinking!

It was the beginning of the end, I just didn't know. By then I had walked away from my PhD, I just couldn't do it. I was embarrassed and a mess, I couldn't spend five minutes with myself, I could barely function sober, so I threw myself into 12-step meetings. I made the choice to once again stop my meds, because the particular 12-step meeting I went to introduced me to someone who insisted I should. For the guts of three years, I binged on pills and moved only between my bed and meetings and occasionally to collect my child from school. On the good days.

That is when I hit another 'rock bottom'. Suicidal and sober. WTF!. That wasn't supposed to happen. I was supposed to be sober, happy, joyous and free! I was done. I packed my child some bags and waited until the midterm break, sent her to my mother's and sat down to kill myself.

And (I swear, this actually happened) a friend knocked on my door. Someone who I knew who struggled with addiction and also struggled with their mental health but was managing both for a few years now and when I opened the door I just burst into tears and told her my plans. A week later I'm in the local psychiatric hospital and have signed up to complete a six-week day programme my friend recommended as she had done the same thing many years ago.

I came off my meds but this time under guidance and with a purpose that maybe, finally, they could give me the right diagnosis and meds and I would finally be ok. I stayed on that program for 10 weeks instead of six. I thought I needed it, and so did they. I received a new diagnosis, one I knew was right. I started on new medications. It was not an easy or simple journey. I spent another year or two binging on pills occasionally but slowly things started to balance out. I started counselling and went every week for two straight years. Damn, that was painful.

Then Dad died. My world collapsed. Broken and alone, my father died. And I swore, by his bed that night, I would not let my daughter watch me die like that. I then swallowed a handful of pills every night for a week. I remember so clearly still, by the Friday of the following week after Dad died at 5 a.m. in the morning sitting in my bed thinking I have to change this, I will die like him. I have to change this or kill myself. So, I did something I hadn't done in nearly 10 years. I applied for a job! And by lunchtime that day, I had done the interview and got the bloody thing. Part-time but doing something I could do and I felt made a difference. Slowly again things got ok. I went to work 19 hours a week on a welfare

scheme. I started getting other support. I made new friends in a new 12-step program, who had struggled with the same stuff I had, I kept going and then one
day I was all of a sudden 1 month clean, then, three months, then six, then a year.
Then three years!

And life got better! I met someone. Someone good, and kind who believed in
me. I started working that 12-step programme, I took my meds consistently and
as directed. I kept my doctor's appointments. I got a sponsor and I got honest.
Then at 35, I got my first big girl job. I started working with homeless people.
I felt useful. I felt maybe I can do for these people what I couldn't do for Dad.
And that is where I learned about Dual Diagnosis. It's also where I learned that
Dual Diagnosis is just about the hardest condition to get help for. I started to
recognise myself in the homeless people I worked with. I became hopeful and
grateful. I knew the only difference between me and them was pure luck. I had,
after all, briefly been where they were. And as I began to understand them, I
begun to understand me. And as I began to understand me, I began to have some
control over my life, over myself. I watched other addicts with debilitating mental
health issues get turned away from psychiatric services who refused to treat them.
They were constantly told, *'get clean, then we will help you'*. Or *'we won't help
you because you're an addict you're not mentally ill'*. For some reason, psychiatric
services in my experience seem to think if you're an addict you can't be mentally
ill, or at least that's the message they sent out to me and in my work with others.
I knew because I saw in those I worked with exactly what I'd experienced all my
life. They were addicts, they were using, but they were legitimately struggling with
their mental health too. I couldn't get clean until I got help for my head. And I
knew that if they had only gotten a chance to get the same help maybe they could
survive too.

I have seen many addicts die, in my personal life and my work life. I battled
with my own soul as I watched and they couldn't get help. They couldn't even see
what I did, what had freed me. Realising my own experience as someone struggling with a Dual Diagnosis finally gave me the understanding, I needed to figure
out that I could get well. That I could be both an addict and mentally ill and that
for me and maybe others, there was a simple answer in treating both concurrently.
With a Dual Diagnosis it's my experience you can't get *'well'* without working on
both, together. I wasn't an addict who needed to get clean. I wasn't a lunatic who
would never function. I was a whole person who happened to be both and if I
addressed both in equal measure I could be ok.

Then I got really well! Work took over. I got married. My partner believed in
me. I got a better job. I made good money. I became a better person. I had goals. I
could see my own potential. And then I got high. Three years of hard work and I
got high. I got a toothache around the same time I was going through some pretty
heavy bullying. I started to blame myself. There's something wrong with me. I
am the reason I am bullied. How am I here again? I started to isolate. I stopped
talking to friends. I got a toothache, so I bought some Solpadine. It helped. A
year later I was in Spain bouncing around chemists trying to get codeine over the
counter. Six months later I broke. The bullying was out of hand I was trying to
look like I was coping, and I broke. I cried to my husband and told him what I was

doing. I told him I needed to go to a psych ward. I then knew I needed to tell my daughter. She was now 16. We sat down with her. I told her how I felt. I told her my plan to get well, and she said '*have you seen how much Solpadine you have?*'. I managed to say '*what!*'. She said she knew I had a pack in my car, a pack in my bag, a pack in my locker and a pack in the medicine cabinet. She asked if I knew how much of it I was taking? FUCK!.

I think then it hit us all. I didn't need a psych ward. I needed to stop using. Because if I stopped using, I had some hope of managing my mental health. Of managing my life. I am now just over three years without a mind-altering substance in my body. I take my meds to treat my mental health regularly and as prescribed. I only take paracetamol or ibuprofen if I have pain.

I talk, I work the same programme that saved my life the last time. I got honest with my doctor. And I am clean, like really clean. Not clean but using pills, or clean but making excuses. But clean and using nothing and living honestly. But this time I do it knowing what I am, knowing who I am and knowing what I need to do to treat it and stay well. Knowing that what I am is an addict in recovery with a mental illness and I need to take care of both to be the person I want to be. It seems so simple now. It's not without its struggles I have to manage my thinking, maintain awareness of how what I think about myself and the world can do me real damage and I have to be super vigilant in looking at myself and my behaviour. I have to take my meds. Everyday. At the same time. But man do I take them willingly and with gratitude now.

I wish now that back then, when I was a teenager, someone had seen it and told me that dual diagnosis was a legitimate condition, all of its own. I wish I had known I wasn't an addict who couldn't ever stop or a lunatic who couldn't be helped. That I didn't have to define myself in opposition to other parts of me. And that I didn't have to be just one or the other. That I didn't have to use to get away from myself. That who I was, was in fact a consequence of both those things but not only these things.

It was only in knowing what dual diagnosis was, that managing me and my life became possible at all. And now I am not just those two things, I no longer define myself by them, I am so much more. I am a good mother. I am a hard worker. I am a kind person. I am an empathetic friend. I am lazy. I can get angry and mean. I sometimes buy chocolate, hide it and eat it alone in the middle of the night. I sometimes go to bed for two days and hide. Sometimes I lie about the tiniest and most meaningless of things. But I am ok. It's not all perfect. On bad days my first thought is still '*I want to die*'. And I have come to terms with that being my default position that I will probably have to live with but today I know I really don't want to die. It's BS. It's old patterns of thinking that take time to change. Today I know I am not my thinking and what I think doesn't define who I am. I define who I am and I am so lucky to have had the chance to figure that out. I have watched too many people die for never having had the chance to get help, to be understood, to understand. People are complex and solutions to our problems need to be complex too. No pill will fix me, no programme will fix me, no counsellor, no psychiatrist, no substance or person. But if I work on both, if I respond to my mental health needs and my addiction needs, if I do these two things together then I have a chance to fix myself.

Chapter 20

My New Beginning, Owning My One Precious Life

Kate Byrne

This is my story of recovery, and of how I took my life from chaos to calm. I was diagnosed as a Dual Diagnosis case when I sought help in 2018. This means I suffered from depression and a dependency issue, a bit like the chicken and the egg question, it is irrelevant to me which came first, all I know is they were a powerful intoxicating burden to carry. I was voluntarily admitted to a residential facility, much to my disgust, as I felt I didn't really need that much help. I would have preferred a magic spell or pill to make the changes. But there is no quick fix for addiction. My cry for help was after many years of being treated with medication for depression. This time things were different, I self-referred to my G.P. explaining that I felt I was dependent on a glass or three of wine every evening. It was something I had tried to reduce or control via abstinence, but I just couldn't manage to resist alcohol. It had a hold over me. My G.P. was wonderfully understanding and so kind, she had known me for years and was surprised with my request for a referral to St. Patrick's Hospital. It is essential that you can ask for help, Doctors treat all ailments, some visible and more invisible. They never judge you and are only too happy to help.

The Formative Years

My story begins when I first had an alcoholic drink at the age of 18 or 19. I never drank in my teens as I was a rule follower, eager to please. I accepted that alcohol wasn't for kids and didn't touch it until I was of age. That first drink tasted horrible, but the effects were astounding. My awkwardness left me, I was no longer conscious that everyone might be watching and judging me. I was able to appear confident and enjoy the social events I had to attend. I was able to feel part of the gang. Unfortunately, this comfort was a false pretence, over the next seven or eight years, I would drink whenever I attended a social event. Frequently when I awoke in the morning, I would realise I didn't remember getting home, or I would

Different Diagnoses, Similar Experiences:
Narratives of Mental Health, Addiction Recovery and Dual Diagnosis, 149–154
Copyright © 2024 by Kate Byrne
Published under exclusive licence by Emerald Publishing Limited
doi:10.1108/978-1-80455-848-520241020

see dialled numbers in my phone that I had no recollection of speaking with the recipients of my calls. The pattern developed of working Monday to Friday and spending my wages on going out Thursday, Friday and Saturday nights. Frequently I would wake very early after a night out, six or seven am, this would be the norm for me after a night on the tiles. This re-enforced a feeling that everything was ok, wasn't I up early and getting things done?

I enjoyed some years of lessened drinking due to having my own family, breastfeeding and pregnancy meant I didn't drink. My children were my priority, and I was able to reduce and control my drinking in phases. I was enjoying a busy life, full of activities I felt represented being a '*happy parent*'. I see now that this was a pressurised phase, somewhat like a pressure cooker – the lid was going to blow eventually. Sadly, my significant relationship deteriorated. In the past there had been many instances of domestic violence and this had added to my nervous disposition. I felt like I was walking on eggshells all the time. I suffered from increased anxiety and broken sleep. It became impossible to function and to me, the obvious solution was to self-medicate with my old friend, alcohol. It didn't matter if it was beer or wine. Either did the trick, calmed me down and took the edge off things at home. What was once a choice, became habitual. I needed a drink to help me feel calm in the evening, it was my reward while I cooked dinner, my treat when the kids were asleep and my medicine after every violent incident in the home. The most traumatic incident was when I was holding my teething son, who was 18 months old at the time. My partner who also drank excessively wanted to take the baby from me to see if he could stop the crying. A struggle ensued where I was punched in the face. This was a turning point for me. Had I not had a drink on me I felt I could have managed the situation better, I could have prevented the violence or at least I could have fled and sought help. There was a guilty feeling that if I sought help, I wouldn't be believed, or I would have been blamed in some way by the authorities or my family. I was a functioning alcoholic and I realised if I wanted to get out of this dark pit I found myself in, then something had to change.

First Steps to Recovery

On the 9th of July 2019, I entered St Edmundsbury Hospital, I felt great shame and desperation at the state I found myself in. I was painfully aware that this was a last resort for me, I had tried and failed to control my drinking on many occasions. I needed support to find the strength and courage to tackle this problem for once and for all. I knew deep down that I couldn't do this on my own. I had observed loved ones in my extended circle decline into chronic alcoholism. I felt if I did not seek help, then this was a real possibility for me too. I had completed questionnaires on the Health Service Executive (HSE) website which confirmed I had a problem with alcohol consumption. I felt that if a hospital stay with professional intervention wasn't to work then my fate would be to waste away in a blur of chaos, isolation and loneliness. I must add here, that many family members and friends thought I did not need help, this was for two reasons. Firstly, no one knew the full extent of my drinking, secondly, some felt that it was ok to drink every day. This is important to note, I knew I needed help. As hard as it is to admit to yourself that you have a problem, it is even harder to convince others you have a problem. You are the expert on this, if things don't feel right then they aren't right.

Inner Turmoil

My life had become a maze of scrambling thoughts, every day I was preoccupied with drinking or not drinking. Guilt and shame were the strongest feelings I endured, when I did succumb to having a drink. My gut told me I shouldn't drink, but there was a relief when I took that first sip. The relief would then reduce and the guilt and shame increased, almost in similar proportion to the drink lowering in the glass.

In the dark recesses of my mind, there was a voice telling me I was ok, I didn't have a problem with drink. Sure, I was Irish, didn't we all drink? Weren't the Irish known all around the world for like a drink? I had three children, a full-time job, a violent relationship in the home... What else could I be expected to do but drink. I could justify my drinking if I chose to, but the reality was I knew this was not the life I wanted to live. This voice, I was afraid of it at first. As I got stronger in my recovery, I started to get angry when this voice would speak negative thoughts to me. I liken this voice to a demon that lives within me, it undermined my confidence, caused me to worry about my ability to stay sober. Undermining my progress, negating the improvements I had made, belittling the relationships I had repaired. This voice I can liken to the devil on my shoulder, a changeling, encouraging you to give up and have a drink. Sometimes I think of it as a cheating lover who says they will never let you down, urging you to return to their loving arms. Telling you everything will be ok, but the reality is you are much better off now without them. You just have to realise that everything will be the same as it was before if you return to this lover, the empty promises, the hurt, the shame and the guilt.

I look at my life now and it bears no resemblance to the stressful, chaotic, mere existence I was enduring until I entered the hospital. I fully engaged with the services, begrudgingly at first. Attending daily classes and lectures was an essential part of the process. I met with my Addiction Counsellor Suzan, a person I disliked immediately as she challenged my behaviour. Hitting a nerve (with a sledgehammer) when she asked if I was emotionally available for my children. I could lie to Susan and say yes, I was, but I couldn't lie to myself. This question cut me to the core. We are great friends now, I have forgiven her directness, in fact, I am extremely grateful for it, as it jolted me into the reality of the situation. I resented that conversation so much for a few days, I moaned to my peers at every opportunity. But the fact was undeniable, I had not been emotionally available for my children, my family or friends or even myself. I had pushed down my feelings so much and buried them beneath a layer of distractions and alcohol. This was a breakthrough moment and a huge relief to realise I could and would change the direction of my life. The most important line I heard while an inpatient was from a fellow alcoholic who had relapsed a few times and was again trying to get sober and stay sober. He said, of sobriety…

> '*You have got to want it more than anything Kate, more than anything else, because without it you lose everything*'

The more I said this line to myself, I realised it was true. If I could stay sober for a day, it was just a matter of repeating that the following day. Sounds simple, but it was the most difficult thing I have ever succeeded in doing properly. I used every tool available to me to get sober. This included an inpatient stay for seven weeks, while released home for a weekend I was met with a house full of alcohol. This was a huge challenge for me, it scared me. But this taught me that I could and would encounter challenges and most importantly I was able to resist the temptation of alcohol if I remembered my core values. I wasn't to be free from the scourge of addiction. Each week other peers and friends returned to the hospital having relapsed. I was so happy to walk back through the doors of the hospital knowing I had stayed sober. This incident also told me; that I did not have support at home. The abuser was happier to have me drinking, it gave him power over me and made me more vulnerable. I decided over the seven weeks stay that in order to save myself I had to love myself for who I was. I accepted myself fully, acknowledging the child within and the life experiences I had gone through. I had a long road ahead of me, but I was proving to myself on a daily basis that this was the life I wanted, no drama and no chaos.

If You Don't Want to Fall Out of the Bed, Get into the Middle of It!

After my stay in the hospital, I attended 12-step meetings in my locality, three or four times a week. I was very lucky to have a variety of meetings to pick from. Once I even attended a meeting delivered in Polish, I explained that I just needed to feel the power of the rooms that evening, and I was welcome to stay. I am not religious at all, but for me, the higher power was nature, the power and beauty of the world we live in and the love of my ancestors. I imagined my ancestors rooting for me, showering me with love and wishing me well. I was a secretary at meetings, made tea and coffee and was always available to help with running the meetings. I felt such love and acceptance in these rooms it was amazing. I also attended step down (a support group), this was a weekly session in the hospital. I travelled one and a half hours each way to make this session – each week I saw familiar faces, sometimes there would be a relapse and we would miss our friends, hoping they would be back soon. This served as a reminder of how fragile our recovery is. I also attended a self-compassion course run by the hospital's psychology department; this was a great support. I learned to lower the volume on the negative voice, to quieten the devil on my shoulder and to love myself back to wellness.

A Fresh Start

Within six months of returning home, the threatening behaviour was worsening. There was a growing resentment towards me and my sobriety. I was increasingly afraid for my safety and the safety of my eldest daughter from a previous relationship. Things got so bad I had to get a safety order and leave the family home. Unfortunately, this coincided with the COVID-19 pandemic hitting Ireland. All refuges and hostels were full, I was homeless with three children. I had to move back to my parent's house, it was a tough time but we were safe, happy and loving towards each other. That was all that mattered. In June 2020, I secured a rental property, returned to work full-time and enrolled in a university course in Adult Education to start in September. I home-schooled my two younger boys, aged 5 and 8. This was a difficult time, but at no time did I feel like my sobriety was at risk. I kept in touch with my counsellor and made sure to check in with her and attend meetings if I felt the need to.

I enjoyed learning online and looked forward to my weekly class, I was enjoying the comradery and friendship without meeting in person. I successfully completed three certificates in the last two years and graduated with a Diploma in Social Science this year. I was accompanied by my father and son, who were both so proud, as was I. I have achieved so much, through adversity.

Looking after myself has been a skill I have had to learn, AA [Alcoholic Anonymous] meetings were the start. These are no longer a big part of my life, but I dip in and out as I feel the need, or just to remind myself of where I once was. I swim in the sea as often as possible; a wetsuit is required at this time of the year but it is my time to have some peace and quiet. I do yoga once a week, I find it relaxes my body and allows me some quiet time. I walk regularly. I have lost weight and I am happy with my figure for the first time in my life. I realised that I needed to slow down and allow myself to be off duty sometimes. Gone are the days where I rush around doing things for others and taking no time for myself. If I am tired after work, I do a set it and forget it dinner – turn the oven on, put frozen food in and set the timer!

There are some changes I made that will stay with me forever.

- I no longer walk down the alcohol aisle in the supermarket, I have no business there.
- I drive to every event I attend; it allows me to leave when I want.
- I don't offer lifts to others in advance, as you can end up staying on to give the person a lift home, even though you want to get the hell out of there!
- I don't have alcohol in my home, again no business there.
- I tell people I am in recovery; it stops the asking *'are you having a drink?'* It also allows them to ask me questions – there are many people struggling, and it might give them strength to see me doing ok.
- Keep learning, learning new things gives me joy so I started a Masters this year. I never thought I would achieve a Certificate or Diploma but now I believe I can do anything I put my mind to as I have overcome greater challenges in life.

- Be yourself, you are perfect the way you are. I pierced my nose and got tattoos at 46! No one cares!! It gives me joy.
- Be active, use it or lose it. I abused my body for so long, I have to look after it now.
- Spread joy and kindness, do good where I can. I will never know the troubles in another's life, but it is good to be kind.
- Find your tribe-you will know them when you meet them, they will love you just the way you are!

Life is great now; I feel love and joy every day. I keep a gratitude journal each evening and this has helped me to reflect on the good in my life. Things have been difficult at times, it can be lonely, but I don't have the chaos I had before, so everything is manageable. The chaos that came from alcohol addiction was frightening, the energy and mental stress involved in hiding it is unbelievable and so physically and mentally draining. I am free to live my life, free from guilt, free from pain. Those around me are genuinely happy for me, I can accept their love knowing I am worthy of it. This is so wonderful, as before I struggled to allow myself to be loved. I am human, I have flaws, but I don't stop working on improving myself.

Recovery is possible, stay strong!!

Chapter 21

To Hell and Back

Anonymous

Introduction

Remembering back to my past, I can safely say that I had what I can only assume to be a normal childhood. I played sports and I had a few friends. I was well-behaved, and I progressed greatly in school. I suppose if I was categorising myself during my school years, I would probably be in the nerd category. Unfortunately, just being placed in that category brought its own problems. I quickly became the victim of bullies. Reflecting on my schooldays, without a doubt, the bullying I received was a very mild dose. In saying that, it still impacted on me. I vividly remember on one occasion the thought of committing suicide just to escape from it. To this day I cannot remember exactly what age I was when I had these suicidal thoughts, but I know I was in primary school, therefore, I was under 12 years old.

Now I know, I said that I had a normal enough childhood, but back then I thought everyone at some stage got bullied. I thought it was normal. I thought it was just part of growing up. The lesson I took from my childhood experiences is that to have a happy life, it is necessary to fit in, no matter what the cost. Unfortunately, it was with this lesson that I went down a treacherous road, a road that I thought I could not return from.

Fitting in

I was 21 years old when I finally met people who I enjoyed being around, who accepted me for the person I was... well for the person I portrayed myself to be [fun, lively, up for the craic and mad]. Unfortunately, in the group, a few people took white [Cocaine] and fast [Speed/Amphetamine]. To be honest, it didn't really bother me for a while, but after some time, I decided to take a line fast. Granted, when I made the devastating decision, I was highly intoxicated from alcohol, but I knew what I was doing. I remember thinking that unless I took something, they wouldn't want to hang around with me. I couldn't bare having that thought turn into a reality, so in order to fit in and continue to be accepted, I took my first line of speed. This was the first step down the rocky road to hell.

Different Diagnoses, Similar Experiences:
Narratives of Mental Health, Addiction Recovery and Dual Diagnosis, 155–157
Copyright © 2024 by Anonymous
Published under exclusive licence by Emerald Publishing Limited
doi:10.1108/978-1-80455-848-520241021

Rocky Road to Hell

If only I could say that one line would do and I don't need anymore, how beautiful that would sound. Instead of the sneaky and silent hold that I call addiction.

It started with the impression that it was a bit of fun. What harm could it do? Just snort drugs one night a week. One night of drugs a week seems manageable? How wrong I was. One night led to two nights, two led to three and so on. In the height of my addiction, I was snorting eight [3.5 grams] of cocaine a day. This was equivalent to €1750 a week. I drained all my savings that I had (€40,000), plus my yearly salary of €25,000 for 6 years, and when all my money was gone, I owed €10,000 in drug debts to dealers. Even then I couldn't accept that I had an addiction problem. I was lucky that I had a family who gave me the money. To make matters worse, I got arrested multiple times for drug-related offences, but I refused to stop drugs as I thought it could not get any worse.

Don't Fool Yourself

If I could give any advice, it would be that no matter how impossible it may seem, when drugs are involved, it can always get worse. So don't fool yourself by saying that it can't. The only limit is death. Let me tell you how every aspect of my life got worse. Through my continued addiction, while high, I put myself in a disastrous position where I left myself open and vulnerable. In turn, I was preyed upon and blackmailed, all due to my addiction. I had no money; therefore, I could not give what was demanded from me. I was publicly destroyed, humiliated, and ruined on social media. I lost everything else that I had, my friends, my self-respect, my self-confidence and much more. I didn't want to live anymore, there was no way out of it. I was hopeless in the search for a solution after this emotional abuse.

My Mind

It was at this moment; that I became aware of the meaning of depression and anxiety. Sleepless nights dominated me, constantly worried of what tomorrow would bring. The simplest task of going to the shop was an internal struggle that felt impossible. The fear of being seen was unbearable. I didn't want to leave the house. Even to eat at the dinner table made me sick. I was ashamed and hopeless. Suicidal thoughts were a constant, everyday occurrence. The only thing that eased the pain was to continue taking drugs as a form of self-medication. As Gabor Mate states *'The question is not why the addiction? But why the pain?'*.

The Way Out

In the summer of 2022, I decided I needed help. Using this as my last resort before suicide, I spent 60 days in residential treatment. I was put onto the dual diagnosis programme. Being on this programme not only dealt with my addiction but also dealt with my mental health. Within this programme, they had to strip the addiction before getting to my mental health issues, but in the end, they both got the attention they needed. Between increasing my education on the issues that I faced and simply listening to other people's stories in the famous smoking area within the facility, I started to feel normal, less frightened, and more accepted. Most importantly, I was understood. I felt that I had a purpose in life and that I deserved to live a life full of peace and happiness.

By being on this programme, I was able to construct a recovery plan that tackled all my issues. Between medication, councillors, psychologists, and support groups, I can start to live a happy and fulfilled life. Thanks to the dual diagnosis programme I found a way out, and I learned to survive.

Difficult Roads Leads to Beautiful Destinations

Now six months into sobriety, life has opened so many new doors for me. The chance to upskill myself and to have fun on a daily basis is an opportunity that I grab with both hands. Being in recovery has its own difficult times and it is hard at times when dealing with depression, anxiety and paranoia, not to take the easy way out and return to drugs. But the fear of losing everything I now have is too scary for me to turn back to drugs. Being an uncle for the first time, meeting new friends, going on day trips to scenic areas all over Ireland with my brother and simply being trusted and being able to buy things that I want without the fear of my bank card being rejected, are all privileges that I have got in my recovery. All these privileges along with being able to see a future deters me everyday from using.

Chapter 22

A Place to Be

Laura Hardiman

When I was 12, I drilled a hole in my head and filled it with bad ideas about myself. It was as if I woke up one day feeling like a terrible person, with a sense that nothing was ever going to be ok ever again. The doctors called it depression, and with that my life took on a different shape. I stepped onto the conveyor belt of the mental health services. It is hard to put a coherent timeline to these years, and hard to find the words to explain the experience. What I can say is that in describing one experience, I am in many ways describing them all. I became very familiar with waiting rooms, the ones with the yellow walls and ticking clocks branded with the name of a popular antidepressant. I'd sit there for as long as it took because appointment times didn't seem to matter. I'd sit there for 1 hour to be seen for 10 minutes, by a different doctor than the last one, and the one before that. During their introductions, I'd try to bear the weight of the disappointment at this stranger and the knowledge that by the next time they may be gone too. I'd wonder at myself for ever being so stupid to have expected any different. I'd wonder over and over why they couldn't review my file before calling me in, but I'd never say it. Rate your mood from 1 to 10 and promise not to kill yourself. That was about the gist of it.

As the years went on, I started to feel like the personification of that '*square peg round hole*' analogy. I could puff myself up and I could shrink myself down, always ending up with a feeling that I was too much or too little, and sometimes like I had no shape at all. Like the difference between seeing your reflection in a mirror or in a window. That is how little I felt seen by the doctors, not surprising given it was how little I could manage to show off myself, just an outline. I can only remember fragments of these experiences now; my memories are just outlining too. It is like trying to recall details of a dream, like it has become a memory of a memory. I say this not only because it is really sad feeling holes where large pockets of your life should be, but also because I often feel like a fraud talking about what I hardly remember. What I do remember is the pain and just how unbearable the world inside me could be. I dealt with this by hurting myself, self-harm became my first addiction. I learned that pain had to be visible, it had to

Different Diagnoses, Similar Experiences:
Narratives of Mental Health, Addiction Recovery and Dual Diagnosis, 159–163
Copyright © 2024 by Laura Hardiman
Published under exclusive licence by Emerald Publishing Limited
doi:10.1108/978-1-80455-848-520241022

be proven and justifiable. The cuts on my body were one of the ways I learned to communicate when I was desperate. Diagnosis and symptoms gave me a lens to understand myself, there was no such thing as my personality, and medication was the only real answer. It was essentially like showing up to A&E with a broken arm for 10 years and not questioning why I just kept getting it re-plastered.

For a number of years, my home environment became very difficult and unpredictable, and I didn't feel safe in school either. I didn't feel safe anywhere, especially inside my own head. Rather than talk too much about all that, I am telling you about the beginning, because I see now how it created a certain kind of foundation for how I operated in the world. You can be hopeless even when you don't know you are and I definitely was. I had spent half my life in services offering support yet I had never learned how to receive it. I didn't have the tools, the awareness or the trust needed to be vulnerable. I was broken and it seemed I would stay that way. I felt monstrous, like something was missing inside of me.

I wasn't so sure what to think when I was told I was an addict. Drugs gave me a sense of stillness, I could finally exhale. I can't say if I went through the contortions of addiction so I could be anyone but myself, or if it was the only time I felt I could be me. Both are really sad, and both were the only solutions I had come up with. A short few years of this solution, I found myself back home with my parents. I was overwhelmed by the very idea of functioning; a day's worth of resilience was often depleted just from getting out of bed. My appetite was so far away that trying to eat was like being invited to sit down to a bowl of plastic. I had to build up a list of go-to foods that felt most manageable, as if I had somehow aged backwards. It started with a banana, and my mam saying

'*One bite at a time…we're going to sit here and face this one bite at a time*'.

We laugh about it now, but the level of responsibility I had to place back on my parents is not lost on me. It's strange to know that there was a version of me that got overwhelmed by the steps involved in preparing and eating a meal.

One morning shortly after moving home, I had a moment of what felt like clarity. The proverbial mask slipped, the veil fell, and I saw myself. I saw my life for what it was, I saw who I was, and who I wasn't. The reality of it all made me feel like I was being buried alive. The holes in my head had grown over the years and once I started to take the drugs away they felt bigger than ever. I felt I could not survive without finding something in its place. By that afternoon I was in A&E with my dad who held me together as the hours passed. During one of my many trips to the bathroom, I stopped and looked in the mirror for a long while before making a deal with myself. I told the mirror that I would give it everything I had. I would get honest, the type of honesty that is painful. I would wrench my heart and my mind open in an attempt to find something that could work. More importantly, I would start to hold myself accountable. If after all this I still wanted to die, then I vowed, I could kill myself. I was eventually seen later that day by the psychiatrist who was, to put it lightly, unhelpful. That didn't matter though, I had found some part of myself during those hours. I was willing to change. I was willing to find a balance between help from myself and help from others. Years previous, after a suicide attempt my dad had said to me

'you don't want to die, you just want to be out of pain'.

It was time to get out of pain. This in many ways, is the exact moment I entered recovery.

If I were to create a map of my recovery and put a pin down for each important pit stop, all roads would lead to peer support. When I began attending addiction counselling I was advised to try out an NA meeting which I ended up attending several times a week for two years. The meetings gave me something to do, somewhere to be, and someone to talk to. The rooms were filled with people who were willing to share the darker corners of themselves and sit with me in mine. I thought recovery was about becoming someone new, something better than what I was. I started to see that it was also about returning to yourself, to parts of you that were lost and forgotten. NA gave this gift to me, beginning and returning. During this time, I also started a programme of dialectical behaviour therapy (DBT). This came out of a short conversation with a nurse and a subsequent referral for psychology. I note this because I want to highlight the impact people can have on you and the trajectory of your life. Even a brief encounter can stay with you when you feel understood, and when people give you their time and presence.

DBT comprised of a weekly therapy session, skills group and homework practices. So just like NA this gave me something to do, somewhere to be, and someone to talk to. Sure enough, I was in a bubble of mental health, but my days were again beginning to find routine and meaning, I had a focus and a bit of purpose. DBT helped me to make sense of everything that had happened, particularly inside my own head. I didn't realise it, but I think I had waited a long time for someone to say to me that given the circumstances, what I was doing made sense. While also offering skills and a different way to understand and manage things. I was blessed to work with my DBT therapist and experience a therapeutic relationship that gave me hope. I had carried so much hurt and fear towards mental health services and those working in it and had been caught in that disempowered way of thinking. My experience with the DBT programme and therapist was very healing for my relationship with myself, and how I related to others. I really saw how I had been stuck in the identity of a helpless child. The gift of DBT was the possibility of hope.

Another form of help and support that thankfully required much less thinking and talking was exercise. My dad kindly bought me a gym pass along with one for himself so I didn't have to go alone. I wobbled around the gym for a while and without much thought or reason gravitated towards running. The 'one bite at a time' approach served me well, 30-second intervals on the treadmill grew into hours on the roads. Running taught me so much about how I understand perseverance, motivation, confidence, when to listen to my head and when to ignore it. Ironically, it gave me a sense of stillness inside me that I had spent my life seeking through anyone and anything around me. I embraced the silence, the boredom, and the solitude of the long distances. I learned to really value my ability to just be with myself. Getting out of my head and into my body allowed me to connect with all the good in me, and take off the heavy winter coat of self-judgement, stigma and shame. This was the gift of running, finding peace within myself.

After two years of recovery being my full-time job, I decided to gradually make some big changes to my routine. I discharged myself from mental health services, I left NA and I went back to work. None of these were spontaneous decisions and they were all things I discussed at length with my biggest supporters. I had started to feel like the cage of mental health and addiction had been replaced with a cage of recovery. A bigger cage with room for others sure, but a cage nonetheless. I had this feeling that I needed to be more than my recovery, and my life needed to be more than a series of things I did to support my health. When I commit I really commit, and I can often do things at 110%, so I was feeling like I had recovery burnout. Leaving services after 13 years was a victory for me, it just felt right. Realising NA was no longer serving me and deciding to leave was empowering. I gave myself the gift of self-trust, the joy of relaxing in life and taking things a little less seriously. A close friend wisely said to me that it's important to get off the personal development train every so often. I learned to reap the rewards of the work done before moving on to the next phase of growth. I think this is paramount to a sustainable recovery, it has to be enjoyable and uniquely meaningful, and not always so hard. I started to realise the importance of being flexible with my needs, and allowing my definition of recovery to be changeable, always evolving over time. I stopped seeking constant answers or solutions and felt freedom in knowing I didn't need them. I stopped pathologising every feeling, every thought, and every emotional response. I stopped saying things like *'that's the addict in me'*.

I was drawn to the informal way of giving and receiving support within NA, the learning and encouragement within the DBT skills group, and the more genuine approach of DBT therapy. I came to understand the difference between help and support, and the noticeable difference in the impact it had on me. Before we finished, my DBT therapist mentioned the recovery college and thought I would resonate with the concept behind it. I began attending workshops and finding ways to get involved. I loved the idea of lived experience being understood as a source of knowledge, and so I applied for the Peer Support course at Dublin City University (DCU). The course really helped me to ground the idea of the illness story versus the recovery story. The diagnoses and the addiction are the story, and the human experience underneath all that is where the learning and an ability to relate to others comes from. I see it as the experience of the experience. Another door opened for me when I was linked with an online recovery community called *'Better Together'*, through one of the recovery educators. I joined with the hopes of enriching my placement experience during the confines of COVID-19 and subsequently found a home for myself along the way. To date, no experience matches the respect, and genuine opportunity to realise my own skills and strengths, as the experience I have had with *'Better Together'*. For the first time, I could appreciate what it means and what it feels like to be part of a community. I could see the power in a type of care and support where there is no beginning and no end to when someone is receiving it, and when someone is giving it. And so, one of the most valuable gifts I got here, is the gift of connection.

At the time of writing, I am shortly approaching six years in recovery, roughly speaking. I can't say I count it anymore and I can't even be sure of an exact appropriate date. I don't mark it by the reduction of a series of symptoms, or the abstinence from a substance. I mark it as an era when I decided to change my life for the better, and no matter what has happened since, I have continued to do that. I work as an expert with experience on the national DBT training team, a peer support worker, and I am still very involved with '*Better Together*'. I have a full life and I can connect with my place in it. I have two very close friends who made so much effort to reconnect with me shortly after I moved home. They invited me into their life and gave me the time it took to feel capable of inviting them into mine. I was with them on the day I realised I no longer wanted to die, I finally wanted to be alive. They are a blessing in my life. By now it is evident I have two endlessly supportive parents who I can never repay, and yet they never make me feel like I need to. I personally would not have survived without these people. They gift me with belonging, every day.

I can never regain the years lost, and there are days I wish I found life easier. I don't like to think that all learning has to come through pain and suffering, and yet I am so blessed and grateful to have found my own way of making it all worthwhile. I truly empathise with those who have not been given as many opportunities, and who are not surrounded by as much support as I am. I want to acknowledge the strength of people who continue to push on despite this, and I hope for everyone to eventually find and receive their own version of gifts.

I can say that recovery is beautiful, freeing, possible and it is. I can say that recovery is difficult, painful, scary, and it is. For me, recovery is a lifestyle and it is also a way of being. This is recovery, a seed inside of me that is always there. Sometimes so small I have to go looking for it, fearful I have lost it and yet somehow always hopeful. I need only to feed it and absorb the light shining out of everyone around me. Connect, connect, and connect. It can be a close friend, the postman, or yourself. Everyone has something worthy inside of them, something that shoots right out of them when they open themselves to another. Now it grows out of me too, wrapping around the people I love, who love me. Communities.

My recovery is about everyone. It is a nod to the patience, generosity, forgiveness and love of friends, family and everyone in between. It starts with the banana, the gym pass, the meetings and the endless cups of coffee at the kitchen table with a listening ear that hears the same problem over and over. People are amazing.

This is recovery, a home inside yourself, full of rooms for everyone to be themselves in.

Chapter 23

A Version of Me

Amy Ryan

It's so hard to describe the period that led to my recovery that I usually simplify it with 'the time in hospital'. It wasn't my first time in a psychiatric hospital, to say the least, but it was the first time I had attempted to end my life. I would describe the experience as a desperate attempt. It was certainly not 'a cry for help'. I had intended to die because I simply could not see any hope, any future or any end to my suffering. I had given up on myself. I felt I couldn't take the pain of life anymore. I was so alone. I had insufferably surrounded myself with friends upon friends all my life to fill the gaping lack of love in my life.

I came from a very abusive family home. Abuse is usually categorised and I can tick all the boxes. Alcoholism was described as 'fond of a drink' in the 1990s, and hidden from the outside world at all costs. I could tell endless stories of the shame and embarrassment of having a violent, alcoholic, abusive parent in small-town Ireland, but what hurts the most is how I was ignored in the midst of it. By everyone. I was a quiet, creative and studious child. The panic attacks were extremely visible, but no one helped. Children backed away and watched with fear as I gasped for air. Teachers sometimes rubbed my back or gave me a brown bag. No one asked me what was wrong. No one cared enough to give me a hug and tell me they would help. I was alone.

The panic attacks and stress rashes were the first visible signs when I was six-years-old. I learned to hide away my pain and grew very sociable, outgoing and outwardly confident as the years went on. As a teenager, I self-harmed my way through puberty. I fought hard to bandage the torture that it was to live inside my mind. I lived with endless, recurring nightmares which was a black figure screaming incessantly. That dream was my life. Shrill, piercing cries inside my mind while I battled to continue the facade of a bright, bubbly teen enjoying her youth. That screaming never stopped until I started using in university. Alcohol and marijuana were numbing, allowing some peace from the endless stream of anxiety, secrets and agony.

I could tell you about the rich and fulfilling life I had while I suffered. I could tell you about the countries I travelled to and all the degrees and courses I completed.

Different Diagnoses, Similar Experiences:
Narratives of Mental Health, Addiction Recovery and Dual Diagnosis, 165–169
Copyright © 2024 by Amy Ryan
Published under exclusive licence by Emerald Publishing Limited
doi:10.1108/978-1-80455-848-520241023

I did that for a long time to justify my use. I 'deserved' to let loose because I was so productive and hard-working. I was highly functioning, until I wasn't. I lost everything in one fell swoop on the other side of the world, right in the middle of the pandemic. My life changed forever in Hong Kong.

'You will never live a normal life if you don't give up drink and drugs', said the psychiatrist while I lay in the hospital bed. It sank in for the first time. I had come so close to death, five millimetres to be exact, that I was considered a miracle by the doctors, nurses and health care workers. I knew it was time to try something new. I sat for six weeks in the hospital bed with nothing and no one to entertain me. The attempt had not killed me, but awoke the fighter in me. I fought to learn how to walk again, to have appropriate care and to recover. The first time I looked in the mirror, I was shocked. I will never forget the pale, broken woman who stood before me. Forever scarred.

After a transfer to the psychiatric ward, I found a treatment centre. I had no idea what to expect and there was limited information to access online. I was confirmed to have a place and discharged from the hospital to go there the following week. For one reason or another, I had to wait two months to get there and that was one of the hardest times in my life trying to stay sober. I felt that I deserved to have one last blowout before I went in but I couldn't because I had no one who would support that. I remember the night before I was due to go in, I bought a bottle of 'Tsang' and parked up inconspicuously. I called my friend who told me it might stop from getting into treatment. I poured the bottle out after one sip. I was disgusted and hated my friend for having some sense.

My time in treatment was the best and worst thing I have ever done. My denial was so strong, that I spent endless conversations arguing why I wasn't an addict. I threatened to leave several times. I threw tantrums and called for managers, I wasn't an easy resident to deal with. I have always been strong-willed and demanding, and these qualities were magnified in a confined space where I was supposed to comply and do as I was told. I disliked almost everyone and spent most of my time writing alone in the corner of the room. I refused to crochet, gossip, find a love interest or open up in the groups. I trusted no one until I met Aisling and Joy. Then began a wonderful journey of opening up, growing and releasing, together. They were my first 'recovery friends'. I spoke for the first time about the sexual abuse I had suffered as a child and subsequent sexual assaults. I never got the hang of freely opening up in groups and I didn't cry away my pain. Those five months were just a bubble for me to realise that I could live without numbing it. I began to see that it was possible. I had hope.

With encouragement from the workers in the treatment centre, I went to a transition house. I didn't last. It was too restricted and after five months, I was ready to start my life again. I left in a dramatic fashion after I refused to do another meeting that day and I was told I wasn't allowed to go swimming because 'it wasn't fair on the other girls'. I went home for about six months, started working online and threw myself into Narcotics Anonymous in my locality. I was drawn to the pain in those rooms for a time, feeling comfort in the sense that I wasn't alone and there was great support in those meetings. However, I found that the regimented nature of the recovery programme didn't quite fit for me.

I couldn't click with a sponsor, I couldn't meditate and I found chairing a meeting re-traumatising.

I searched elsewhere. I found an addiction studies course which I might as well have eaten whole. I craved to understand the disease as much as I could and I found it liberating sharing my experience with others doing the course. I was encouraged to become a tutor, something which I am still working to achieve. I needed that kind of support at the time and my tutor was amazing. It reignited my passion for learning and began to forge a new path for me. That is where I learned about 'Better Together', a support group for people in all forms of recovery, be that mental health and/or addiction. I felt an immediate connection and I remember crying the first time I shared, which was and still is a rare occurrence for me. I felt at home with others who knew what 'struggle' meant but the meetings were relaxed, joyful and heart-wrenching, all wrapped into one.

'Better Together' became my daily support network, as well as my growing number of recovery friends. Early recovery was tough. The emotional pain of the past was now acknowledged, and I was aware. Aware of what had happened, aware of mistakes I had made and pain I had caused, aware of my emotions. I had no idea what to do with all this awareness or where to start. Every day seemed to bring new challenges and my familiar coping mechanisms did not serve me any further. I talked over my problems in the groups, with my therapist and with my recovery friends. My friends and I learned from each other, consoled and counselled each other. It was hard.

In the middle of all this, I broke my ankle. This was a triggering event for my family and I was told I had two weeks to leave home. With nowhere to turn, I left for a sober house with a charity who aided homelessness. I was homeless again, but this time I was sober. I felt the pain more intensely than before and leaned on my supports to hold my hand. I didn't cry then; I wailed. The pain of experiencing this, while I was trying my hardest to be better, was immense.

The sober house was challenging. The other person in the house wasn't sober. I lived in fear and my anxiety soared. I kept working, I kept going. I lost a lot of weight because I couldn't eat, distracted by fear. I felt so alone again but my friends were phenomenal. They got me through. After about six weeks there, I finally found a flat, living with my best friend. It was perfect. I had managed to find somewhere in a short space of time, in the middle of a housing crisis. I still live there now, one year later and I'm very happy. I enjoy the anonymity of city life and I have met good people there. I have found a home in my heart in Ireland. There is no more chaos in my life, which is as much a miracle as the fact that I'm still alive.

I was shocked that I remained sober through a difficult living situation but nothing prepared me for the shock of failure in the form of a 'slip'. To me, the vocabulary was important when it happened and I insisted on correcting anyone who called it a relapse. What it is called is no longer important but what I learned was the important factor. Like many of us, I need to make mistakes in order to learn. It is an unfortunate condition of being human because we tend to put ourselves under pressure to be perfect, even though life is imperfect. I felt like a failure because I returned to old coping mechanisms to deal with an awful situation. However, looking back now I see that it was just an attempt to regulate my emotions. It didn't work for me and I saw that a life of alcohol being my solution wasn't what I wanted anymore. I stopped counting my months of sobriety and decided to continue with all the learning I had behind me. I'm so proud to say that I'm over two years in recovery and I don't feel any guilt that I didn't let a slip make me go back to day one again. I think counting the days, weeks, months and years only matters if you can separate from that and count how many relationships you have fostered, how many times you've been there for yourself and how many things you have achieved. I'm grateful now for my achievements and my mistakes too.

Following the relapse, I found myself reaching to all corners to distract my mind. I love to be busy, but my life sometimes feels like an endless schedule. I suddenly found myself working tirelessly. I began to crumble quickly. My mental health was suffering. What saved me was that I could spot the signs and '*took action*'. Burnout can happen rapidly and the signs weren't plain to anyone except me, until I got to the point where I had to take a week off work and could barely get out of bed. Then, it was more obvious. However, I had known that my wellbeing was slipping by small signs like struggling to get up and forgetfulness. I wasn't my usual self. I reached out to the mental health services for support. After a difficult night in A&E, I had hope because I was referred to the home-base team. However, I was quickly told that I wasn't 'bad enough' to avail of these services, in spite of my history and diagnosis. Aside from that, I was worried because I didn't have family support. Instead of wallowing in the lack of, I took action and reached out to those who I knew could help. 'Have you eaten or showered today?' This was helpful. Sometimes overwhelm blindsides with the simplest of tasks.

I've learned so much about myself on this journey and one of the hardest lessons is that I can't do life on my own. I've always beaten myself up for leaning on anyone, even though I always did. That endless battle inside my mind has quietened by simply accepting that I need others to survive. I may not need who I would have expected to need; knowing where to turn is the most important on this path. I have 'ainm chairde' who accept me for who I am. They respect what I am doing in living a sober life and they support me in watching for signs that my mental health is slipping. I have learned through my experiences that I can't do it alone and I'm comfortable with that now.

I've stopped trying to escape. Throughout my recovery, I have made plans to move elsewhere. Unconsciously, I have tried so hard to run as far away as I can. My eyes twinkle at the sight of an opportunity, but something has always kept me here. I have a good life in Ireland now. I have the opportunity to work in mental health, which is something I always dreamed of. I volunteer my time helping others who have similar struggles and I teach. I'm busy, trying to make the world a better place in my own small way. When I really struggle to find gratitude, I find that I am reminded to be grateful that I am alive, that I'm here to live another day and work towards being the best that I can be. I'm also grateful that I have room and a car. It's these things that make everything possible because I know what it is like to live without them.

The story of my recovery is not a simple one. I didn't just stop drinking and have a better life. My recovery has been a winding road of mistakes and mourning the life I have left behind. I've left people behind too and I miss them all the time. I get tired of trying so hard sometimes, but then I remember what addiction led me to. I still get flashbacks about my 'time in hospital'. I don't know if that will ever stop. My therapist tells me that I'm traumatised by what I did. How can you traumatise yourself? That person who tried to die wasn't me; I'm scared of needles, I don't like to see blood, I'm not violent in any sense, except I like watching Tarantino movies. I can't watch them anymore. So, who am I now?

That's what I'm trying to rediscover. Every moment of every day, I try. That's the best I can do.

Chapter 24

Maybe One Day...

James (Jimmy) Lewis

Pleaze App Ltd., Ireland

For as long as I can remember, I've never been happy. In fact, I don't know what happiness is nor do a lot of people. Some people think it's an emotion or feeling. Personally, I just think it's a state of calmness, peace of mind with an ability to deal with whatever life throws at you. Unfortunately, I've never been there...yet. From about the age of 10, which is as far as my memory goes, I was an unhappy child and kept to myself. I have always felt uncomfortable in this world, as if I wasn't made for it or I was a mistake. For various reasons, but we'll get to that. Around this time, I was suicidal but unaware. I was actually unaware of how I was feeling and thinking because I didn't know any better or couldn't understand it. My mother had found a drawing I had done, depicting me hanging from a tree. But why? Why was I feeling like this? What happened? Could it have been the fact that I was horrifically bullied? Maybe because my father wasn't around? Or was I just born like this? It's a billion-dollar question, and still, to this day, no one has been able to answer it. I mean, they've all had their say, but all have a different take on why I am the way I am. I must mention that I've been to them all, therapists, psychiatrists, psychologists, addiction counsellors, psychiatric hospitals, rehabilitation clinics, nutritionists, neuroscientists and the list goes on.

My story is somewhat of a unique one. I've been diagnosed with nearly every mental illness under the sun, tried pretty much every treatment available and there isn't much I haven't seen or heard. At the time of writing this, I'm 27 years of age. You might get the impression that I'm almost boasting or proud of how horrible it is to be me. This is just my truth. After being bullied for a number of years, I subconsciously created a new identity and character. See, I thought I was the problem. The little quiet scared child was disliked by everyone, so I thought I had to change. Welcome the new me. Jimmy – the outgoing, funny, *'crazy'* character who is always the centre of attention. When I moved to school at the age of 13, it worked. Jimmy was finally accepted.

Different Diagnoses, Similar Experiences:
Narratives of Mental Health, Addiction Recovery and Dual Diagnosis, 171–174
Copyright © 2024 by James (Jimmy) Lewis
Published under exclusive licence by Emerald Publishing Limited
doi:10.1108/978-1-80455-848-520241024

I had my first drink at the age of 10, Tia Maria – bizarre, I know. I didn't make anything of it really. That changed when I decided to have another go at 13. Instantly, it was what I was looking for all along. That uncomfortable feeling vanished and everything felt better. The drinking wasn't that often throughout my early teens, but I specifically remember saying to myself around the age of 15, '*I absolutely love alcohol*'. Deep inside, I knew what was to come.

You can get away with it in your teens, you're young, having the '*craic*', it's what everyone else's doing. I stuck out like a sore thumb on alcohol, it changed me. I was bananas really. Extreme and wild. There wasn't a party that I didn't take all my clothes off or fought to be the centre of attention. There was a little bit of weed here and there but nothing crazy. It wasn't until I was 18 and on my sixth-year holiday in Magaluf where I decided to numb the pain further – MDMA, otherwise known as Ecstasy. Around this time, I managed to get myself into my first relationship. I was madly in love. The problem was my drinking was heavily impacting it. I was reckless, sometimes cheating, disappearing for days, etc. I remember the day like it was yesterday when it all changed. It was like someone flipped a switch in my brain. Lights off, pure darkness. A deep, depression had begun with suicidal thoughts flowing frequently. This was the first time I was consciously aware that something was terribly wrong.

Fast forward a year and the relationship was over. I haven't been the same since. Heartbreak is my Achilles heel. It sends my whole world crashing down. Hello cocaine, I need help, I can't cope anymore. From this point, it is a consistent downward spiral. I thought I was hitting rock bottom, but it just kept going further down, down and down. I started running away from my problems, thinking it would solve everything. I just brought them with and everywhere I went I would create a mess of everything. Australia, Thailand, South Africa, various counties in Ireland – the same story. Wanting to die and endless alcohol, drug, gambling and sex abuse. There are quite a few attempts on my life around this period. To this day, I'm baffled as to how I'm still alive. I could go on endlessly with insane stories, but let's talk about the history of the treatment I've received.

At the odd time in my early life, my mother would send me to someone to talk to, but I had no idea what was going on. My teachers would constantly request for me to be tested for ADHD [Attention Deficit Hyperactivity Disorder]. I don't blame them; I was ridiculously disruptive and eventually wasn't allowed to many classes. – '*Mr. Lewis, you don't have ADHD*'. Interesting... I had a complete mental breakdown during my holiday in Thailand. My mother had to come out to collect me and bring me home. Within a couple of days, I was admitted to a psychiatric hospital. The diagnosis continues, '*It looks like Dual-Diagnosis, Borderline personality disorder, ADD* [Attention Deficit Disorder]*, addiction*'. I didn't last very long in this hospital, the doctors were constantly on holiday, the programmes were pointless and to be honest I was too young to want help.

We call this period the dark winter when I was released. How would I describe this, let's just say I became a scary person. I start seeing a therapist once a week, we start unravelling my childhood. '*I would probably say unipolar, possibly bipolar but definitely an addict*'. I should mention I'm on medication at this point, an antidepressant. That was about as far as I would go. I didn't believe in medication, why numb everything rather than work through it? Never mind the side effects... During this time, different therapists and doctors would tell me '*You're a young, good-looking guy, you have your whole life ahead of you*' and '*It's time to stop being the sick one in the family, time to grow up and be a man*'. How on earth do they think this will in anyway help me? It wasn't until I was caught for drink driving a year or two later that I decided to go to a psychiatrist again. He doesn't say a word for two hours and just types on a computer as I'm telling my story all over again for the 100th time. '*Let me get you some more pills*'. Lamotrigine, a mood stabiliser. No change.

I head off to South Africa to see if I can get some help there. Over the course of six months, I worked intensely with a psychologist. The verdict? Bipolar. Double the dose of Lamotrigine. I'm feeling somewhat better you could say so I decided to come to home. I'm a little over six months sober now and falling in love again for the first time in four years. When I'm in a relationship or in love, it's like all my wounds instantly heal. Unfortunately, I relapse again, start cutting myself and have a very near miss on a suicide attempt. Straight into rehab. This was probably the best and worst five weeks of my life. The greatest foundation for recovery someone could ask for. They pulled out everything in a matter of weeks that others couldn't in years. I now understood why I have to numb the pain – living in reality is too painful.

Sober and in love. I couldn't ask for much more. Too good to be true? Shot to the Achilles heel, oh no it's coming. This time, like never before. I can't go on any-more. My whole life has been filled with pain and suffering. '*Why should I go on? For who? For what? So, you don't have to suffer when I kill myself? No more*'. I enter the psychiatric hospital on my hands and knees, this is it. My one last chance at life. Over the course of about eight months, I had five separate admissions. I could no longer live in the real world. I actually contemplated never leaving. The usual happened - endless therapies, diagnosis, medications and you name it. On my final admission, I openly declared that this was my final try, do whatever you want. My health insurance is running out in a few weeks and I will be taking my life if noth-ing works. I had planned the whole thing and to be honest, I was looking forward to it all finally being over.

As per usual, they come up with nothing. My parents decide to intervene. The googling starts. '*New treatments for suicidal thoughts*' etc. We found a place out-side Ireland that does Ketamine assisted therapy, rTMS [repetitive Transcranial Magnetic Stimulation] and neurofeedback training. The couple of weeks wait to get there were extremely lucky. The suicidal thoughts were so bad, I couldn't even hang on until I got there. During these weeks, I start seeing another doctor who wanted to treat me through supplements. I also visited a doctor specialising in neuroscience whose take on me is that I had a traumatic brain injury from drug and alcohol abuse. He claims that I also have PTSD and that the ketamine treat-ment I will receive will be great for me. On top of that, my testosterone levels are low and TRT [Testosterone Replacement Therapy] was recommended.

The night before treatment, I'm in my hotel room and contemplating to jump off the balcony. Fast forward 2 weeks, 6 ketamine infusions, 10 rTMS sessions with 10 neurofeedback tests, and I'm crying my eyes out. But not because I'm sad. For the first time in my life, I wanted to live. I saw a way through, the light you could say. I was excited about my future. Since that day, a little over a year ago, life hasn't been all that bad. It doesn't require a lot for me to be '*happy*', as the bar is so low. If I wake up and feel okay, I'm blessed. Although, I do still have bad times, suicidal thoughts, and bouts of depression. I get a ketamine treatment every six months as a '*top up*' dose. I did relapse after two and a half years of sobriety, unfortunately. After a long but fun year, I'm back on the straight and narrow doing what's suggested.

My life probably isn't going to be an inspirational story of how I overcome depression, suicide, and addiction. This is a lifelong journey. Who knows, maybe one day it will all click, and I'll be happy like the rest of you. So, what's my advice? Well, if you're struggling with your mental health, get a second opinion or a tenth. We are highly complex humans and there is more than one approach to treating you. In regard to addiction, I only know one solution. That is to follow the principles of Alcohol, Narcotics, Cocaine, Gambling or Sex and Love Anonymous. The quicker you get help, the quicker you will recover. I'll leave you with one final tip. Learn to master your mind and emotions as this pretty much creates your reality. The rest will come together naturally.

Part 5

The Fusion of Experiences

Chapter 25

Fusing Experiences, Reflexive Thematic Analysis

Michael John Norton[a] and Oliver John Cullen[b]

[a]*HSE Office of Mental Health Engagement and Recovery, Ireland*
[b]*HSE Mental Health Services, Ireland*

Abstract

This chapter presents the results of a process of reflexive thematic analysis. It highlights the recovery journeys of those with mental health, addiction and dual diagnosis challenge. In doing so, a number of similarities occurred. These included beginning in a place of trauma, working to cope with the trauma, seeking help from services, peer support, relapse and finally fully embracing recovery in one's own life. A number of differentials were also identified, including additional steps in the mental health recovery journey along with the title of various phases of recovery. The chapter ends with an acknowledgement of these similarities and differentials which the following chapter can then utilise as a basis for making recommendations to policy, practice and the users of services themselves.

Keywords: Recovery; trauma; substance use; psychopathology; relapse

25.1. Introduction

As documented in Chapter 3: 'Recovery in Mental Health, Addiction and Dual Diagnosis' recovery is observed as an abstract concept. However, it is also a non-linear journey taken by individuals which is unique to them as they walk through the bumpy road that is life (Jacob, 2015). This chapter aims to identify the similar concepts, characteristics or phases that make up the recovery journeys

Different Diagnoses, Similar Experiences:
Narratives of Mental Health, Addiction Recovery and Dual Diagnosis, 177–206
Copyright © 2024 by Michael John Norton and Oliver John Cullen
Published under exclusive licence by Emerald Publishing Limited
doi:10.1108/978-1-80455-848-520241025

of individuals with mental health, addiction, and dual diagnosis challenge. To identify these concepts, characteristics and/or phases, a process of reflexive thematic analysis of the previous 18 narratives will occur. In Section 25.2, the theoretical and practical applications of Braun and Clarke's (2006, 2019, 2022) reflexive thematic analysis will be explored as the model used to analyse these 18 narratives. After which, the results of this process will be documented. In Section 25.3, the results of the process of reflexive thematic analysis as it pertains to mental health will be documented. This is followed by the results of the addiction reflexive thematic analysis [Section 25.4] and the dual diagnosis reflexive thematic analysis [Section 25.5]. Once this phase is completed, a discussion of such similarities in concepts, characteristics and phases will occur in Section 25.6. Finally, Section 25.6 will conclude this chapter by summarising what has been found as a process of reflexive thematic analysis and set up for Chapter 26: 'Recommendations as it Relates to Policy, Practice and Service Users'. The process of reflexive thematic analysis is now presented.

25.2. Braun and Clarke Reflexive Thematic Analysis

Reflexive thematic analysis is a methodological process developed by Virginia Braun and Victoria Clarke through their seminal 2006 work: 'Using thematic analysis in psychology.' It provides an accessible and theoretical flexibility to the analysis of qualitative research (Braun & Clarke, 2006). In order to perform reflexive thematic analysis, the researcher/reviewer must become familiar with the data – in our case narratives, through multiple readings of the same (Norton, 2021). From which a set of initial codes are generated and later combined to form themes and sub-themes (Norton & Flynn, 2021). Such themes and sub-themes are, over time, revised, adjusted and refined by both MJN and OJC until a final list of themes and sub-themes are agreed (Norton, 2021). Any disputes were teased out with both reviewers/researchers until a consensus was reached. Additionally, the reflexivity aspect of this approach comes from the reviewers/researcher engagement with their own subjectivities and preconceived ideas as they pertain to the narratives of the 18 contributors. This is then supported by a process of reflection (Braun & Clarke, 2022; Norton, 2021; Norton & Flynn, 2021). What follows is the results of this process of reflexive thematic analysis.

25.3. Mental Health

From the reflexive thematic analysis of Chapters 7–12, a number of themes and sub-themes came together to construct a journey of recovery for mental health. This journey begins in the trauma phase where trauma occurs along a timeline, made more possible through a list of compounding factors. This leads to a nose dive that brings the individual to a suicidal state where reality is questioned. In an attempt by the physical body to save the entire self, the body enters a freeze like state known as an epiphany of stasis. At this juncture, help is sought, a diagnosis and medication are given and the person begins to grieve for the former self, which eventually leads to the promised land of recovery where the individual regains their life and returns to what makes life meaningful and joyful for them. This process is now discussed.

25.3.1. Trauma

The person's recovery journey does not start at the point of diagnosis. According to the six mental health narratives, gathered as part of this text, the process begins through experiencing some level of trauma in life. Here, trauma is generically described as a 'normal reaction to a set of abnormal circumstances' [JL]. These abnormal circumstances define the traumatic experience and are generically categorised under typologies. This thinking behind the origins of mental health challenges is becoming far more dominant within mental health discourse, with Michaela stating that, in her professional and personal opinion 'mental health challenges a[re a] response to trauma, abuse, grief, inequality, discrimination, poverty, stress and isolation' amongst other factors. However, the onset of these experiences, differs from person to person. Added to this, these six narratives have found that there are several precursors or compounding factors that act as catalysts to traumatic experiences. In essence, these are tell-tale signs that a person is more vulnerable to a traumatic experience. The theme of trauma has two sub-themes: the onset of trauma and compounding factors. These sub-themes reflect this discussion and are presented both figuratively and in text in Fig. 25.1.

25.3.1.1. The Onset of Trauma

The mental health narratives noted various time points for the onset of trauma. Most often, the first trauma experienced by individuals came from the supposed safety of the family home. Anonymous described their formative years as being in 'a house that had domestic violence, psychological, physical and emotional abuse'. For others, the onset of trauma occurred later on in life. The Eternal Student noted how they were 'bullied in [their] teenage years [and i]n college'. The abuse can also occur in adulthood, whether that is through a romantic

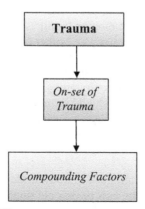

Fig. 25.1.   The Theme of Trauma.

relationship – domestic, or a once off encounter – sexual. Regardless of when the onset of trauma occurred, the resulting impact is similar for the victim of trauma. Anonymous eloquently describes themselves after experiencing a traumatic event as 'a ticking time bomb' motivated by self-loathing, loss of confidence and a 'feel[ing of] hatred for the people who' [TES] carried out the traumatic act. For those who experienced sexual trauma, there was a noticeable 'feeling of dread [that] smothered [the individual as] memories of the events ... [comes] flooding back' [LMcG]. Unique to those with sexual abuse, the legal route of prosecuting the offender serves as a re-traumatisation of the act. For instance, L. McGowan described how her body, as part of legal proceedings, was re-violated as a 'physician took photos of [her] naked body for "evidence"' [LMcG]. Although, these experiences re-visit and haunt the receiver of trauma, for 'the most part a few minutes after hearing about it, life moves on and [the victims are] barely give[n] it a second thought' [LMcG].

25.3.1.2. Compounding Factors

As noted above, traumatic experiences can occur at any point in the life cycle. However, for the six contributors to the mental health narratives, the onset of trauma occurred in childhood/adolescence and early adulthood. However, for trauma to occur, there needs to be a number of confounding or precursive factors that make an individual more prone to the said experience. For Michaela, the first compounding factor originates early in childhood in the supposed safety of the family unit. She describes how her 'formative years were [shaped by her] immediate family [being] fractured by alcohol and boarding school, immigration [and the] absence of [the] wider family circle'. This differs to L. McGowan, whose confounding factor came after the traumatic event in the form of a lack of justice/support. For L. McGowan, despite re-traumatising herself again for the purpose of pursuing legal action, she was informed that '[her] case ... would not be heard in court'. Confounding factors can occur along the lifespan. One such factor is death. From the six narratives reviewed under mental health, two types of death were seen as particular precursors for trauma – sudden death and suicide. Anon described how she discovered that her Mum was 'in hospital for weeks. [with] cancer' This lasted 'a few short months [until] ... she was dead'. In addition to this, Anon also lost in 'the same week ... 2 other family members ... and a friend' Michaela, on the other hand, described her 'big sister, whom [she] adored, killed herself [at the age of] 18'. Regardless of the factors that made individuals prone to trauma, the reactions to these confounding factors were similar. L. McGowan described how she 'felt so small, childlike, and alone'. Whilst Michaela 'was in shock and couldn't grieve'. In Michaela's case particularly, a sense of deja vu occurred where she found herself forming her own fractured family in young adulthood:

> I became pregnant I continued to study, while also working to support myself and my son as a 19 year old single parent. [MMcD]

25.3.2. Nose Dive

Once the traumatic experience takes place, a nose dive occurs where the individual is often filled with a wave of unwanted emotions. This is further entrenched through the sensitivities that each individual is genetically predisposed to. As a result of the negative emotions caused by the trauma and or/their compounding factors, and their genetically predisposed sensitive nature, the individual concerned becomes consumed by negative self-talk which can lead to a sense of hopelessness. Such hopelessness, depending on the nature of the emotional response to trauma, can lead to one of two outcomes: suicidal ideation and/or a lack of reality. Fig. 25.2 visually illustrates these events within the individual's recovery journey.

25.3.2.1. Sensitivity

Sensitivities describe the 'highly intuitive, empathetic and sensitive' [MMcD] nature of the six contributors to mental health in this text. It describes how, due to their unique personality – which is genetically predisposed – individuals are more sensitive to life than others. Such sensitivity can be positive, but in this scenario, can also have negative connotations. For example, Andrew identified how his sensitivities led him to 'hear terrifying noises … [that] soon turned into short and sharp voices telling [him to "shut up!" … how useless [he] was, [and] how [he] should end [his] life'. A similar situation occurred for The Eternal student who 'one night … heard three people talking through the wall, … trying to threaten to come into the house and attack [him]'. As noted by both Andrew and The Eternal Student, their sensitivities made them prone to auditory hallucinations which impacted their daily lives including their ability to 'sleep all night … [and] do [their] job' [TES].

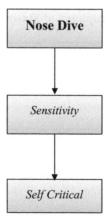

Fig. 25.2.   The Theme of Nose Dive.

25.3.2.2. Self Critical

As a result of these sensitivities, the individual contributors in this text begin a process of negative self-talk which is often critical to the self and portrays the self in a negative light. Michaela describes how she was self-critical because she was 'a perfectionist and high achiever' who was always 'readily accepting responsibility to make things better'. Jenny noted how they felt that they were not 'enough, [they] would never be enough'. Such negative self-talk led to contributors feeling 'a sense of aloneness and "fitting in" rather than belonging' [MMcD]. Such loneliness which resulted from the negative self-talk exhibited above left individuals 'sad, lost, confused, hurt, lonely and utterly, utterly devoid of hope' [JL]. The result of this hopelessness led individuals to one of two outcomes 'ending up in hospital, on suicide watch …' [Anon] or in a space where one 'could not understand what was happening to [them]' [AG], resulting in one questioning their reality:

> I had no idea yet how I had come to this place or what was even real anymore. [JL]

25.3.3. *'Epiphany of Stasis'*

'Epiphany of Stasis' is the third phase of an individual's recovery journey. It is characterised firstly, by a lack of trust in oneself, which leads to isolation and loneliness which then leads to guilt. This guilt overwhelms the individual to the point that they want to end their own life, but in a way that does not want to hurt the feelings of others close to them. This friction in the mind ends up having a somatoform response as the body and mind generally freeze in an attempt to save themselves. This process is visually depicted in Fig. 25.3.

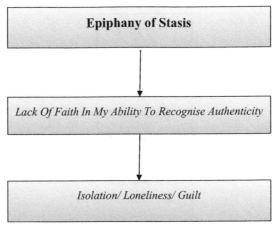

Fig. 25.3.   Epiphany of Stasis.

25.3.3.1. 'Lack of Faith in My Ability to Recognise Authenticity'

Once the person becomes suicidal or loses their sense of reality, the mind can cause the individual to lose 'faith in [their] own ability to recognise authenticity' [JL]. This is a dangerous time for the individual as the loss of faith in their authenticity causes their sense of safety both within themselves and to those around them to be questioned. Andrew depicts this lack of faith in their authenticity and decent into madness in the following quotation:

> Then in July, just two weeks after the birth of our second child, I started hearing and seeing quite distinctly three evil men – the voices were now embodied. They were real [I lost 'insight']. Everywhere I went they seemed to be there – there was no escaping them. They were deriding me, tormenting me, sometimes screaming and shouting and swearing at me. They started performing experiments on me – they implanted maggot-like eggs in my brain, I could feel them hatching, and the alien creatures feasting on my brain. They implanted a micro-chip in my hand in an attempt to try and control me – sending electric shocks up my arm when I didn't do their bidding. They, and those working for them, were trying to steel my thoughts, making me confused and forgetful. The men were also trying to insert their thoughts into my mind. They started to command me to harm some of those around me. They felt like all-powerful, all-knowing, godlike malevolent presences. I was utterly terrified at the thought that I might comply with their demands. [AG]

25.3.3.2. Isolation/Loneliness/Guilt

Through not trusting the safety of the self, one then slowly slips into darkness. Jenny depicts this by stating: 'I slipped away, … though I found myself surrendering completely, pulled in by the shadows while the others took in the sun' [JL]. However, isolation in this context does not mean isolation in a literal sense. Michaela suggests that isolation could involve packing up your life and beginning again somewhere else where else and 'forming new relationships with people who knew nothing of [their] past'. Anon goes one step further to suggest that this isolation can also come from 'dissociation. Being here but being so numb to here that there is no "here"'. Here anon associates this dissociation with the self-destruction and death of the self. Jenny notes that at this point the physical body and the emotional self are engaged in a battle for survival and in the 'organisms' attempt to survive, 'it incapacitated [the self]' [JL].

25.3.4. Diagnosis

From the six mental health narratives in this text, once someone reaches a place of incapacitation, the next step is seeking help from services. However, the

experiences of the contributors of the text tell us that the service is often unhelp-
ful. Due to regulations imposed on the service, the focus seems to be centred on
the patient rather than the person. This focus on the patient means that mental
health services observe the person as a diagnosis and not a real person. As a
result, treatment seemed to centre around medications to reduce symptoms of
mental distress caused by a diagnosis. From the contributors' perspective, this
was ultimately seen as harmful:

> I conclude that diagnosis of mental illness, and subsequent and
> continuous treatment with copious amounts of psychotropic
> drugs was harmful to my mental and physical health. Painful,
> necessary emotions were numbed, so couldn't be processed, and
> healed. [MMcD]

The resulting harm left individuals, like Michaela 'powerless to [the] system'.
Fig. 25.4 visually depicts this aspect of the person's recovery journey.

25.3.4.1. Societal Perspective

Once the person enters the service, there is an expectation that they would be
treated like a human being – with dignity and respect. However, as Jenny reports,
this ends up not being the case as the process, for her, 'felt "patient focussed"'.
Patient focussed in this context refers to being objectified as a diagnosis and not
an actual human being. Jenny goes on to describe how service providers 'looked
so put together, so impersonal and unapproachable' leading her to question the
safety of the services themselves:

> I thought this space was meant to be safe. [JL]

25.3.4.2. Psychopathology

When one focusses on the process of diagnosis itself, the first point of contact is
usually through a 'visit [to a] General Practitioner [GP]' [LMcG]. This consisted
of 'a five minute consultation … resulted in a diagnosis of depression' [MMcD],
'post-traumatic stress disorder [PTSD], anxiety, and hyperarousal' [LMcG] which
leads to 'a follow up appointment and a prescription for psychotropic medication'

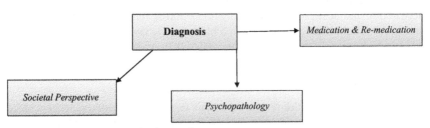

Fig. 25.4.   The Theme of Diagnosis.

[LMcG/MMcD]. Individual contributors were not satisfied with this process as 'no context [was given as] to why [they [fe[lt that] way, no mention of ACEs, trauma, grief, or stressful living conditions' [MMcD]. In addition, there was 'no signposting to practical support or talking therapy. A medical diagnosis with pharmaceutical response was [the]only option' [MMcD]. In fact, the above approach pathologised normal responses to difficult life events as Michaela explains:

> The diagnosis told me that feelings of sadness, anxiety and overwhelm weren't a natural response to difficult life events, because these events hadn't been mentioned. Instead, my emotional response was framed as malfunctioning. This was a physiological issue, a chemical imbalance in my brain that could only be rectified medically, with a chemical cure. [MMcD]

For some contributors, this process made them 'reluctant to seek professional help for their distress because they fear 'just being handed [a] "script"' [MMcD]. For others, they 'leaned into all the supports, medical, mental and otherwise' [Anon] as they felt that the diagnosis 'validat[ed them] after years of just being labelled a drama queen' [Anon]. In seeking help from services, contributors, like Andrew, just wanted 'someone [to] simply sit with [him] and support [him] whilst [he] engaged with' his distressing symptoms. However, the focus here still remained on the system and 'whether this [process] was clinically helpful or not' [AG]. In this way, services lacked the 'human response' [MMcD] contributors required to 'ease their distress. Instead, these people are often [left] on "medication" indefinitely, as their only option ... to tolerate the intolerable' [MMcD].

25.3.4.3. Medication and Remedication

Once individuals were placed on medication, many found that it took time for the therapeutic effects of the same to become established. The Eternal Student highlighted that when he 'was put on medication, [it]took a month to work' [TES]. Once medication reached its therapeutic effects, a number of contributors noted a set of side effects that 'crept up gradually' [MMcD]. Such side effects included 'ma[king] it hard[er] ... to think' [TES], 'gain[ing] a huge amount of weight ... anaesthetised all feelings ... intuition was blunted, and ... creative energy saped' [MMcD]. All of which was not told to the contributor before commencing medication:

> There was no information on side effects, potential harms, or dependency. [MMcD]

Such side effects have a monumental impact on the individual concerned, impacting both their physical, emotional and social health:

> [...] this effected my self-esteem. I had a tremor, itchy skin and constant thirst, this effected my social skills. [MMcD]

Worst still, taking psychotropic medication does not mean that the symptoms of mental distress dissipate. The person can still go on and experience distressing symptoms like The Eternal Student 'hearing critical voices'. When side effects are 'discuss[ed] ... with medical prescribers they [are often] dismissed ... [and the person is] offered ... more drugs to stop [the] body ... reacting to the drugs it was already struggling to process' [MMcD]. Ultimately, by 'numbing the painful feelings, prescription drugs ... robb[ed contributors] of ... natural coping mechanism' [MMcD].

25.3.5. 'Mourning the Self I Used to Be'

Once an individual receives a diagnosis and commences treatment, the individual enters a period of grief where they 'mourning the person [they] used to be' [LMcG]. According to L. McGowan, she mourned by sitting 'on [the] couch in shock and pain ... feeling alone [and]I cr[ying] in a way [she] had never cried before', as she knew 'she was gone and ... wasn't coming back' [LMcG]. After this period of grief, the person becomes a stranger to themselves as a result of the physical, emotional and social impact of treatment, which ultimately results in the silencing of the self. Fig. 25.5 documents visually this process as part of an individual's recovery journey.

25.3.5.1. Stranger to Myself

The mental health challenge and the psychotropic medication used to combat such challenges can have a devastating impact on the individual. For Jenny, this

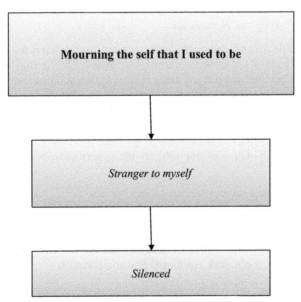

Fig. 25.5.   Mourning the Self I Used to Be.

encompassed a feeling of hopelessness and of death, where 'what little brightness there was left in [her] extinguish[ed]' [JL] to the point that 'the lightness and laughter of [her] neighbours [which] ordinarily would have drawn [her] back to life ... burnt itself out' [JL]. In addition to this, the experiences of trauma and treatment made L. McGowan feel 'like a victim'. All of which 'forced [her] to sit in the company of a stranger – [her]self [as she] did not know who [she] was' [LMcG].

25.3.5.2. Silenced

Due to this now lower identity, individuals with mental health challenges are silenced in some way or another. For L. McGowan, her silencing came from the legal system when her attacker was allowed 'to walk free' [LMcG] and any attempt 'to name him publicly would be an offence and leave [her] open to a potential defamation case' [LMcG]. For Anon, her silencing came from the services in which she was receiving treatment. Anon tells us how 'It was burn't into [her] ... not talk or tell others' about her struggles. When Anon, did reach for help, she felt silenced, 'invalidated and repeatedly dismissed ... by medical teams' [Anon].

25.3.6. *'Promised Land of Recovery'*

It is at this phase that individuals enter 'the promised land of recovery' [JL]. The promised land of recovery is 'so individual that it is hard to write about for fear of invalidating someone else's experiences' [Anon]. However Anon tries to describe what her journey to the promised land of recovery is like for her. Here she likens recovery to:

> a heart machine recorder for my life. Those peaks are like no other, the contentment and celebration of all the work that has led to this point. Those valleys require me to fight minute by minute or daily sometimes and they are dark and unforgiving but there are moments of balance on the incline and decent. One thing it will never be is just 'balanced' because that would be a flat line on a heart monitor if there is a flat line, you are dead. [Anon]

From the six mental health narratives, there are three centralised themes relating to the promised land of recovery: support, 'felt at home with the other crazies' and 'cracks, chips and imperfections highlighted and made more beautiful'. Support documents both the traditional and alternative support mechanisms in place for individuals who have a mental health challenge. One such mechanism that gets further attention is that of peer support under the theme: 'felt at home with the other crazies'. Finally, the process ends with the person finally facing the issues that led to distress, building trust with the self and finally returning to work/career and what gives a person meaning in life. Fig. 25.6 visually illustrates this last part of the recovery journey.

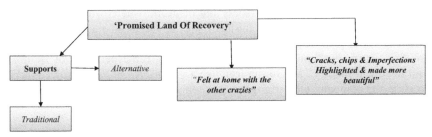

Fig. 25.6.   'Promised Land of Recovery'.

25.3.6.1. Supports

Under support, there are two sub-themes: traditional and alternative. Traditional describes both the safety gained from being in or utilising a mental health service and the disengagement from such services. This is followed by the use of alternative services, where individuals are observed and treated as a whole person, not just a disease that need eradication. These sub-themes are now presented.

25.3.6.1.1. Traditional.   From the contributors who discussed traditional supports, two spoke of the safety that traditional services can bring. According to Jenny, she:

> breathed in and held onto life … breathed out and let go of it. And so it continued, until the love of [her] family, the care of [her] doctor and the guidance of staff in A&E carried [her] to the safety of the psychiatric ward. [JL]

For The Eternal Student, the psychiatric hospital was a mechanism to 'to have some time to reset'. Jenny agrees with this, suggesting that the hospital gave her 'the space and the time, the quiet and the permission to do nothing'. Despite such advantages, the power of psychiatry and the psychiatric ward was sometimes abused to force individuals into compliance as was the case for Andrew:

> I felt coerced back onto Clozapine, with the consultant basically saying that they could use the Mental Health Act unless I complied. [AG]

Along with this, individuals lost faith in services as the 'prescription had only ever increased … indicate[ng] that it wasn't working' [MMcD]. This led individuals, like Michaela, to 'disengage from the mental health system'. The benefits of disengaging were clear in Michaela's scenario as she 'not only accepted, but grown to love [her] authentic self; that free spirited, emotional, empathetic, initiative and nature loving person [she] always was' [MMcD].

25.3.6.1.2. Alternative.   As individuals pulled away from traditional systems, the more reliant they became 'on the psychological techniques' [AG]. For instance, for The Eternal Student, this came in the shape of dialogue with the voices which he learned from attending the Hearing Voices Network:

> One day I told the voices 'I love you' and to my surprise, I heard them say back 'I love you too'... There are groups where you can get help with voices, called the hearing voices network. [TES]

Through the Hearing Voices Network, individuals like Andrew benefitted from 'being around others with similar experiences'. For others, this move away from services led to 'the countryside and [an] immers[ion] ... in nature' [MMcD]. For Michaela, nature:

> [...] reconnected [me] with the raw, hurting version of myself that never had a voice. In solitude, I cried and wailed from the depth of my being, held with acceptance, love and support by other-then-human nature ... I felt, processed and released a lifetime of grief and emotional pain, and I healed. [MMcD]

25.3.6.2. *'Felt at Home with the Other Crazies'*

For those who moved from the support of services to support of peer-led groups, a sense of kinship/community developed between those with similar experiences as Jenny now explains:

> I met people, lovely people, strange, sick troubled, crazy people who felt like me, that something fundamental has been broken in them. [JL]

This community, was an open door, allowing individuals to share 'everything that happened, in great detail, step by step, sometimes for hours at a time. And I did this weekly' [LMcG]. By having this free space to communicate the depth of hurt experienced through life adversity and subsequent mental health challenges, individuals like L. McGowan 'felt empowered ... to turn [her] experiences into something positive' [LMcG]. This is achieved by separating the traumatic event from the learnings achieved from it as Jenny now describes:

> Am I glad I was raped? No. Do I value the experience? No. But the lessons learnt, and the growth I have salvaged from this process of healing? That, I can treasure. Therein lies the gold fault line. And the strength. [JL]

Once this is achieved, those with lived experience begin to realise that their experiences can actually be a source of knowledge that can be used to improve service provision as Andrew now explains.

> Over time, I began to realise that my experiences of 'the men'... were being treated like credentials, like a form of knowledge

and expertise. What I had only thought of as deficits were now being turned into assets, and that I could use some of the darkest moments of my life to make a difference. [AG]

In addition to this realisation, other aspects of life also support the individual to live a life of their own choosing. For Andrew, these factors included his 'amazing church family' and his 'own Christian faith, which [he describes as] a source of hope and help ... even at the darkest time ...' [AG]. Faith as a support was also described by The Eternal Student who found solace in Buddhism:

> Buddhism taught me how to gain more control over my mind by putting in positive thoughts and emotions. The biggest lesson I learned from Buddhism is to try and help others [love] this makes both them and you happy. This lesson greatly helped my recovery. [TES]

Andrew and The Eternal Student both noted family members as another source of aspect of life that positively supported their recovery. For Andrew, it was his 'loving wife' whereas, for The Eternal Student, it was brotherly love as he now describes:

> I remember I shared a bedroom with my younger brother. One night I said there were three people in a car, I can hear the car, I have really good hearing they were going to come into the room and attack me. My brother told me to get into the other bed in the room with him and put his arms around me and said if they come into the house we will fight them. My brother's words filled me with love and courage. Looking back now I know my brother knew there was nobody outside in the car. [TES]

25.3.6.3. *'Cracks, Chips and Imperfections Highlighted and Made More Beautiful'*

Once moved away from services and the above supports were in place individuals were able to accept that they experienced mental health challenges and face their demons. For Jenny, this occurred through the realisation that her 'brain w[as] not sick, [her] spirit w[as] simply broken'. This allowed her to be able 'to say the word "rape" out loud, in relation to myself'. This has an empowering effect, allowing individuals the ability to 'investment in [them]sel[ves] and [their] future well-being' [JL] and 'to right some wrongs and begin the process of rebuilding ... [and] healing' [JL]. This rebuilding includes 'learning boundaries and what [one] do[es] and do[es] not accept' [Anon] and in so doing, regaining trust in the self as Michaela now explains:

> Can you imagine if I had told my psychiatrist that I was getting into the cold sea in winter and had stopped wearing shoes? I touched and talked to trees, listening to what they had to tell me.

I wrote frenzied non-sensical streams of consciousness in the middle of the night. I danced freely whenever I felt the urge to move and shake my body. Without needing to understand why, I tapped my fingertips on my head and face to relieve tension. I tuned into the cycles of the moon and seasons and followed their rhythm. [MMcD]

Once the self is trusted again, other aspects of life then follow suit. For Andrew, Anon and Michaela, this all meant 'returned to work' [Anon], 'but only in a role that … a holistic approach that valued education, self-determination and community connection' [MMcD] and also provided 'some financial stability as a family' [AG].

25.4. Addiction

As occurred in mental health, a reflexive thematic analysis of the addiction chapters (13–18) has also occurred. Once again, the recovery journey here begins at a place of trauma which is experienced in a number of settings and at various time points along the lifecycle. These, yet again, are influenced by a number of compounding factors. This leads to a space we call 'Mind Fucked' where the individual struggles with the impact of trauma. From which, substances are used as a coping mechanism. However, over time, the effects dwindle, relationships break down and the individual finds themselves in a state of crisis. At this point, the individual seeks safety from services, where they break the cycle of addiction, utilise therapeutic supports and those offered naturally through peer support mechanisms. This leads to a place of recovery which non-linear, focusses on the whole person and other positive relationships in the person's life. This ultimately leads to a life worth living. The addiction journey of recovery is now presented.

25.4.1. Trauma

Like within the mental health narratives, the recovery journey of individuals with addiction does not start at the time of diagnosis. Rather it begins with a traumatic event[s] with a series of compounding factors that make an individual more vulnerable to distress from such experiences. The first sub-theme of trauma is typologies of trauma. From the six addiction narratives, there are multiple sources of trauma reaching from the supposed safety of the family through to the aspects that can only occur by others in the community. The second sub-theme follows a similar journey to that present in the compounding factors for mental health. These describe a range of precursors that make individuals more prone to the negative effects of trauma. Fig. 25.7 visually illustrates this theme and its sub-themes.

25.4.1.1. Types

The first type of trauma is trauma that occurs in the supposed safety of the family home. It is termed domestic violence. From the six addiction narratives

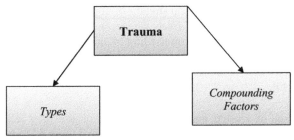

Fig. 25.7.   The Theme of Trauma [Addiction].

in this text, only Arlene and Shay describe domestic violence as part of their recovery journey. However, they are at two different time points. Shay describes how domestic violence invaded his home as a child:

> My parents were arguing and this was becoming more frequent. I remember waking up to shouting things crashing and doors banging. I remember lying in darkness in my bedroom and hearing this going on and waiting for the next loud bang to startle me or the door to burst open. Mam followed by dad shouting. This was becoming more frequent and more physical over the next couple of years. [S]

For Arlene, the onset of domestic violence was more gradual. When she first met her abuser 'he was incredibly handsome, kind, considerate and loving'. However, as the relationship developed the veil slowly fell off to reveal the monster within:

> Gradually, bit by bit all that disappeared, and I became trapped in hell. [A]

For Paul, his childhood experiences were different. He experienced emotional abuse which manifested and created Pauls, the 'scared little kid'. The trauma had such a profound impact on Paul that 'to this day [he still] don't fully understand why' [PG]. In terms of Shay's childhood experiences, on top of the domestic trauma experienced at home, the school presented another, this time psychological trauma in the disguise of bullying, which had a profound impact on him as it made Shay feel 'quite alone'. For Arlene, not only was her partner a source of trauma, but her wider family unit also became another source of trauma when she was raped at the hands of her uncle:

> In 2020 I attended a family funeral ... one of my uncles kept handing me glasses of wine. I don't even know how many I had but these days I was not able to handle it. We had gone to the pub at 3pm and at 6pm I woke up with a bloody nose, a black eye and torn clothing after being raped at the hands of my fathers brother. [A]

25.4.1.2. Compounding Factors

Like the mental health narratives, the addiction narratives provide us with some compounding factors that would increase the likelihood of trauma and the severity of the debilitating effects that come from the experience. Having a member of the family with a mental health or addiction is a compounding factor as John describes:

> I was a sensitive child who was deeply affected by mental health challenges in my family, alcoholism amongst older siblings and occasional domestic violence. [J]

Additionally, the loss of a loved one is another compounding factor. For Shay, the death of his Dad at 52 was 'a big blow [for him] and [he] hit the bottle quite hard after this' as he could not deal with this loss. This differs from Paul, who instead of mourning a person, was feeling guilt over his emerging sexuality:

> So during these years I had also become increasingly aware of my sexuality being opposite to the way I lived my life. No matter how I try to suppress this unwelcome truth the realisation that I was gay began to haunt me .... [PG]

The final compounding factor is isolation. Shay describes how he was 'a lonely child ... [without] any support or someone to comfort [him]'. This sense of pure aloneness was also documented by Paul who tried to 'seek out that state and find comfort in isolation'. The result of these compounding factors is simple, they can 'severe[ly] impact on [ones] mental state of mind and confidence' [S], which Paul suggests are 'some of the character traits that are relevant to people with addiction issues'.

25.4.2. *'Mind Fucked'*

'Mind Fucked' is the second phase of the recovery journey for those in addiction. In essence, it documents the body's reaction to traumatic experiences and the coping mechanisms required to deal with such trauma and its effects. Fig. 25.8 illustrates the theme of 'Mind Fucked' and its associated sub-themes.

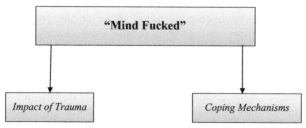

Fig. 25.8.   'Mind Fucked'.

25.4.2.1. Impact of Trauma

Once the traumatic experience occurs, the person's first reaction is 'to feel real anger towards [the perpetrator] ... for what [they were] doing' [A]. As time 'progressed so to did the confusion and turmoil in me, it created anger and resentment, ... [which subsequently caused an] inability to handle life' [PG]. This led to 'fear and always guessing when the next argument or drama would unfold' [J], thereby leading to shame as Shay describes:

> [...] weekends were now filled with him drinking throughout and me spending time alone in the house and hiding my fathers drinking from friends. I was not able to have friends over at this stage because they were starting to notice and I was feeling ashamed. [S]

The shame and fear felt by contributors led to the rise of substance misuse and indeed mental health symptoms such as 'anxiety' which 'made it harder for me to perform daily tasks in life' [MC]. This is adequately described by Shay who experienced similar after smoking weed:

> One night in my Mams in town we had been smoking [weed] and I was at home on my own after and started to feel a bit uneasy in myself. This overwhelming fear and panic started to set in on me and I couldn't calm myself down because I didn't know what was happening to me. [S]

The shame and fear also created a sense of 'paralyzed hopelessness' [J] within individuals. In an attempt to maintain equilibrium, taking substances increased to the stage where social relationships were diminished, financial hardship ensued and 'drugs ... [became] an escape ... in some ways' [J]:

> I got to the stage of active addiction that I had no friends left. I also was left with no car or apartment. No one would talk to me because I was too out of control and I was hanging around with the wrong people, which led me to having run ins with the law on more than one occasion. [JK]

However, in the case of Mark, 'drank more to cope with the stresses of life, ... alcohol [w]as my medicine to keep me going'. However, along with the temporary soothing effect, addiction can also bring people, like Jack, down a slippery road to 'loneliness, isolation, self-loathing and self-destruction'. For John, addiction was a way to express his self-hatred:

> I remember using cocaine in an effort to hurt myself and could not get enough of it to satisfy this desire such was my unease and rejection of myself. [J]

However, such abuse of substances led to more mental anguish as Jack 'urinat[ed] into bottles, because [he] was too paranoid to even go to the bathroom'. Despite this, contributors described still not accepting the fact that they needed help, as Paul now describes:

> Up to the age forty-eight, I was using heroin intermittently … although I was aware my use of drugs was causing problems in my life, I somehow felt that I was in control as the outside stuff, kids, marriage and my career were still somewhat manageable. [PG]

25.4.2.2. Coping Mechanisms

From this point on, the frequency of substance misuse makes the user require it to cope with a multitude of situations. However, it also has several social advantages for the user. Firstly, drug use can 'g[i]ve [the person] … confidence … [and] ma[k] e [them] feel positive, sociable and outward' [J]. According to Paul, they make him 'feel whole, and less afraid and bolstered [his] self-esteem'. Additionally, substance misuse can provide a person with a false sense of belonging 'through risk taking behaviour' [J] with peers. Shay describes how he would steel alcohol to drink with friends down a laneway:

> I would sneak cans out of the house after coming home from the pub with my dad and consume more alcohol with my friends down the lane. [S]

However, despite the initial positive effects of substances, after a while, issues start to arise that become unbearable for the user as Paul and Shay now explain:

> My mental health had gotten so bad that everyday activities were becoming impossible and life in general was becoming unbearable. I was surviving not living. [S]

> Denial, avoidance and using drugs to numb me was becoming less effective and the pain it brought was at times unbearable. [PG]

25.4.3. Seeking Help

As the pain of the initial trauma sets in, individuals begin to reach out to services for help and support. This involves coming out to the fact that you are a user and breaking that cycle of using. In addition, to support this process, the use of peer support and being around those who are experiencing difficulty like you, supported the process of feeling safe within services. Fig. 25.9 illustrates the theme of seeking help and its sub-themes: safety in services and peer support below.

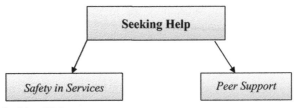

Fig. 25.9.   Seeking Help.

25.4.3.1. Safety in Services

In order to seek safety within services, the first step for individuals is to 'I finally admitted defeat and reach out for help' [PG]. Once this occurs, the services put a number of measures in place to support the individual. For some, this involved a stint of 'residential treatment' [JK], where they received support from a variety of professionals, including counsellors and social workers. Individuals noted catalysts for recovery from these professionals including: 'having [someone] who believed [them] that [they] could do well in recovery and reach [their] goals over time ... helped so much in [their] confidence' [MC]. In addition, such professionals helped 'put into perspective what was happening, what [they] went through and how [their] whole perspective of life had changed over the years of consuming alcohol' [S]. As a result, these treatment mechanisms 'helped [individuals] battle [their] addiction and [put them] on the road to recovery' [JK] as such interventions helped individuals to 'beg[i]n to think that it might be possible for [them] to live a life without drugs' [PG].

25.4.3.2. Peer Support

As part of individuals treatment in residential settings, they are exposed to other people with similar challenges, which provides the individual with 'peace and solace' [JK]. In addition, meeting individuals with similar difficulties provides comfort as the person begins to realise they are not alone on this road as Shay now explains:

> I have met some of the best and courageous people I know in my recovery journey having battled their own demons that I will hold dear to my heart and support in times of need. [S]

25.4.4. 'A Nice Clean Sober Life!'

Through the support of residential treatment, service providers and peers, the individual begins to embrace recovery in their lives. However, recovery is non-linear and involves at times relapse. However, over time, the person begins to find their voice again and enter a life worth living. This life encompasses being honest with oneself and being personally responsible for one's own life. Fig. 25.10 visually illustrates the theme of 'A Nice Clean Sober Life!' and its subsequent sub-themes of In Recovery and 'A Life Worth Living' below.

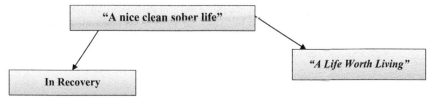

Fig. 25.10. 'A Nice Clean Sober Life!'.

25.4.4.1. In Recovery

The first step towards a nice clean sober life is acceptance that there is a problem that needs addressing. Arlene describes from her experience that after her 'sister begg[ed her] to go into residential treatment ... [she] eventually had a serious chat with [her]self and a look at [her] life [she realised she] needed help [as she] could not do it on [her] own'. It was only after this acceptance that individuals, like Paul, could 'really embraced the help offered there'. However, just because one accepted they needed help, did not mean that this was the end of the battle. Recovery is non-linear and whilst the person enters sobriety, their 'addiction is on the side line doing press ups, sharpening its claws and waiting to sink its jaws [back] into [them] again' [A]. Sometimes, the addiction wins a battle and the person enters a phase of relapse. This can happen at any point in the life cycle from straight after treatment, like in Jack's case, or months later like in Arlene's case.

> [...] I went in for four weeks of treatment ... life was great upon completion of this treatment but it did not last long. I had many issues and challenges ahead and it was all to easy to revert back to using drugs as a means of escaping the reality of my situation. [J]

> Then three months later I was hammered and driving up the road to drink on the road side and driving back. Lunacy! [A]

Regardless of when relapse occurred, the fact is that for many, they would have 'a series of using episodes with gradually diminishing periods of clean time in between' [PG]. However, when the right 'supports [are] in place [the person can] finally really dedicated [themselves] ... to recovery' [S]. As one dedicates themselves to the recovery process, they find 'a voice again' [A] and use it to take back control of their life as Arlene now describes:

> [...] I am in the process of a custody battle. This time the courts are listening to me. [A]

In order to maintain recovery, individuals lean on their natural support mechanisms like family as Paul now describes:

> [...] I in no way want to exclude or under-estimate the power of a loving family in keeping me well and recovering. I am one of the very fortunate people who suffer from addiction problems to still

have a family who loves me, supports me and provides that belonging that I crave as a human but yet turn away from when my head is not right. Somehow my family have been able to see past the sickness and see me. [PG]

At this point, the individual and their family take 'this chance to heal together' [PG]. Only at this juncture, can the individual accept the fact that their addiction is a part of them, but does not define them as Paul now describes:

My addiction is just a part of me, like my sexuality and my work and being a Dad, a friend, and a brother, it will always be a part of me but it does not have to define me, like all parts of me it makes me who I am as a person, and I am proud these days to say my name is Paul. [PG]

25.4.4.2. 'A Life Worth Living'

It is through accepting that the addiction is part of you that one can accept responsibility for their sobriety and wellness. Personal responsibility, according to Mark, includes 'reaching out and trying different supports like peer support groups and engaging in recovery led initiatives such as now writing [a] narrative'. Paul adds to what personal responsibility looks like for him stating: 'its about growing up, taking responsibility, taking ownership of [their] choices and decisions going forward and being accountable for the consequences of those choices'.

25.5. Dual Diagnosis

Finally, we reach the stage of dual diagnosis – the fusion of mental health and addiction challenges. Through reflexive thematic analysis of Chapters 19–24, a journey of recovery has been constructed. Once again, the journey begins in a place of trauma, which is experienced at different points across the lifespan. The typology of which varies from person to person. As a result of the trauma, or of life in general, the person is desperate to find a place in which they belong, which leads them exposed to vulnerabilities and possibly subject to investigation by law enforcement in order to demonstrate to peers that they belong in a certain group. Resulting from this, there is a decent into crisis as substances are used to self-medicate, leading to addiction, self-harm and eventual suicidal ideation. This eventually leads the individual to ask for help, where they are diagnosed and given a prescription for medication. It is not until the individual comes across peers in a similar situation within a peer support group that they accept where they are in life and progress to a place of recovery. At this phase, recovery is seen as non-linear, but is achievable due to factors like family and friends, exercise, viewing the self as a person and not a set of psychopathologies and eventually a return to the self the person wants to be. The process of recovery for dual diagnosis is now presented in more detail below.

25.5.1. Trauma

Like that of mental health and addiction, recovery from a dual diagnosis challenge does not begin at the point of diagnosis. In fact, it begins at the point of a traumatic experience. In the case of Laura, such trauma occurred at the age of twelve as she now describes:

> When I was twelve, I drilled a hole in my head and filled it with bad ideas about myself. It was as if I woke up one day feeling like a terrible person, with a sense that nothing was ever going to be Ok again. [LH]

In terms of traumatic experiences leading to a dual diagnosis, the six narratives for dual diagnosis in this text point to three types of trauma that can lead to such issues later in life: psychological, sexual and domestic. Fig. 25.11 visually highlights the theme of trauma along with its sub-themes below.

25.5.1.1. Psychological Trauma

Psychological trauma, within this part of the text, relates to the impact of bullying on the self. Anon describes how he 'became a victim for bullies ... [during his] school days' [Anon]. He goes on to say that although it 'was a very mild dose ... its still [had an] impact'. For both Anon and Jimmy, the impact of bullying was similar – suicidal ideation:

> I vividly remember on one occasion the thought of committing suicide just to escape from it. [Anon]

> I was suicidal but unaware ... my mother had found a drawing I had done, depicting me hanging from a tree .... [JL]

25.5.1.2. Sexual Trauma

Whilst some contributors suffered psychological trauma, others suffered from sexual abuse. For all contributors effected by this, the sexual assault seemed historic in nature, having 'suffered [it] as a child' [AR]. Regardless of when it occurred, individuals, like Claire, can remember it vividly as she now describes:

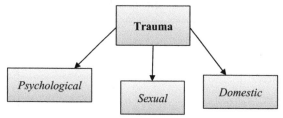

Fig. 25.11.   The Theme of Trauma [Dual Diagnosis].

> [...] they left me there with a guy we kind off, sort off, knew, who lived in the same area we did. Next thing I remember I am on my back, not really able to move or object, on top of his army jacket and that is how I lost my virginity. I found alcohol and sex on the same day, and I would never, ever, be the same again. Now I understand what happened to me as rape. [CF]

As a result of the abuse suffered, despite the fact that it was not the person's fault, they still felt 'shame' [CF] and blamed themselves for the actions of the perpetrator.

25.5.1.3. Domestic Trauma

For the final two contributors, the abuse they suffered was domestic in nature. Although they do not provide examples of such abuse, they do allude to the detrimental impact of the abuse. For Amy, not only did she feel 'shame and embarrassment of having a violent, alcoholic, abusive parent ... but what hurts the most [was]how I was ignored in the midst'. Kate adds to this stating how she 'suffered from increased anxiety'. Eventually, the abuse became severe enough that she became 'increasingly afraid for my safety and the safety of my eldest daughter' leading to 'a safety order and leave the family home' [KB].

25.5.2. 'The Devil on My Shoulder'

'The Devil in My Shoulder' represents the second phase of recovery from dual diagnosis. It is characterised by three sub-phases: [non] acceptance, substance use/misuse and diagnosis. [Non] acceptance describes a phase in life where individuals try their best to fit into a community. This often leads to vulnerabilities that also lead to substance use/misuse as a way to boost confidence and self-medicate from deficiencies in their own lives. As substance misuse increases, this impacts their core relationships which leads to suicidal ideation and self-harm. Fig. 25.12 visually depicts the theme of 'The Devil on my Shoulders' and its sub-themes below.

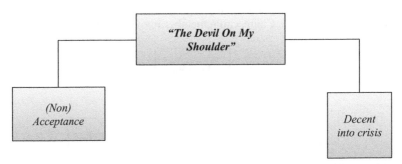

Fig. 25.12.   'The Devil on my Shoulders'.

25.5.2.1. (Non) Acceptance

(Non)acceptance describes the feelings of isolation and the longing to find a place to belong. A number of contributors describe 'creat[ing] a new identity and character' [JL] as they 'felt monstrous, like there was something missing inside …' [LH]. For Jimmy, he felt he was a 'little quiet scared child [who] was disliked by everyone' [JL]. Claire exhibits similar feelings suggesting that for 'as far back as I can, feeling different and lonely and permanently scared' [CF]. In a 'desperate … [attempt] to be loved' [CF] participants felt that they 'had to change' [JL]. This change, according to Anon included taking illicit substances in a desperate bid to fit in:

> I remember thinking that unless I take something, they won't want to hang around with me. I couldn't bare having the thought turn into reality, so in order to fit in and continue to be accepted, I took my first line of speed. [Anon]

This resulted in people 'accept[ing them] for the person [they were] … well for the person [they] portrayed [themselves] to be …' [Anon]. After which, the continuous use of substances led the individuals concerned to be left open to an array of vulnerabilities. In Kate's case, the use of substances empowered her abuser. In Anon's case, it had more dire consequences – destroying himself from the outside in:

> Through my continued addiction, while high, I put myself in a disastrous position where I left myself open and vulnerable. In turn, I was preyed upon and blackmailed … I was publicly destroyed, … I lost everything else that I had, my friends, my self respect, my self confidence and much more. [Anon]

Once these vulnerabilities are exploited, the individual's support mechanism is withdrawn and the individual slips down a rocky road. For Amy, she began to suffer from panic attacks, 'but no one helped … no one asked me what was wrong. No one cared enough to give me a hug and tell me they would help. I was alone' [AR]. To combat loneliness, the individual continues to use substances like 'alcohol and marijuana [to] numb [the pain], allowing [for] some peace from the endless stream of anxiety, secrets and agony' [AR]. In addition, the use of substances eliminated 'th[e] uncomfortable feeling[s] … and [made] everything … better' [JL]. For Laura, drugs also 'gave [her] a sense of stillness, … [which allowed her to] finally exhale'. However, over time, this gradually slipped into a full-blown addiction as Anon now describes:

> It started with the impression that it was a bit of fun. What harm could it do?… I drained all my savings that I had [40K], plus my yearly salary of 25K for six years, and when all my money was gone, I owed 10K in drug debts to dealers. [Anon]

which leads to Anon to be 'arrested multiple times for drug related offences ...' and Jimmy to be 'caught for drink driving'. The decent into addiction also impacted participants' relationships as Jimmy describes:

> Around this time, I managed to get myself into my first relationship. I was madly in love. The problem was my drinking was heavily impacting it. I was reckless, sometimes cheating, disappearing for days etc. [JL]

As a result, in a short period of time, substance went from being a source of confidence and comfort to a mechanism of escapism from the horridness of this world, as Claire now elaborates:

> Using just became the easiest way to escape the pain of being conscious and feeling like I couldn't cope in a complicated world where I had to worry about what others thought of me and where I fit in. Unconscious was always my end goal when I used. [CF]

25.5.2.2. Decent into Crisis

As the addiction continues, the person becomes 'hopeless in the search for a solution' [Anon], which leads to 'endless alcohol, drug, gambling, and sex abuse [and] wanting to die' [JL], as ' [their] whole life [was]filled with pain and suffering' [JL]. This led to 'self-harm[ing behaviour to relieve] ... the torture [of] liv[ing] inside [their] mind' [AR]. Self-harm according to Laura was a way of proving and justifying the pain she was feeling. As such, this was Laura's way of 'communicat[ing] ... I was desperate'. Over time, self-harm resulted in 'quite a few attempts on [their] life' [JL]. However, such attempts came with an epiphany. For Laura, it was 'you don't want to die, you just want to be out of pain'. Whereas for Amy the 'attempt had not killed me, but awoke the fighter in me'.

25.5.3. 'Transformation of Self'

'Transformation of Self' describes the third phase of a person's recovery journey from dual diagnosis challenges. It begins with a diagnosis of a dual diagnosis challenge along with the treatment options available by the traditional system for such challenges. Ultimately, due to these traditional treatment options, participants felt that they received little to no support from services. In fact, it is not until they meet their 'recovery friends' at various meetings that they feel a sense of acceptance over their diagnosis and begin to ride the process of recovery. Fig. 25.13 illustrates the theme 'Transformation of Self' and its sub-themes below.

25.5.3.1. Services

Once participants engaged with the services, the common path was 'receiv[ing] a ... diagnosis ... and ... start[ing] ... medications' [CF]. For Laura, this process

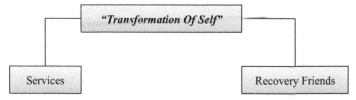

Fig. 25.13. 'Transformation of Self'.

'gave [her] a lens to understand [her]self'. However, for Claire, this process left her 'feeling just as F**ked up as [she] was going in' as she 'went back doing what [she] knew ... drank too much, found other drugs, slept around continue to cut [her] self and ma[de] intermittent attempts to kill [her]self' [CF]. For Laura, she used a metaphor to elaborate on how ridiculous the process was:

> 'It was essentially like showing up to A&E with a broken arm for 10 years and not questioning why I just kept getting it re-plas-tered'. [LH]

As this revolving door scenario continues, support from services dissipated. Jimmy describes how service providers showed a lack of empathy to him whilst he was in active dual diagnosis:

> During this time, different therapists and doctors would tell me "You're a young, good looking guy, you have your whole life ahead of you" and "Its time to stop being the sick one in the family, time to grow up and be a man." How on earth do they think this will in anyway help me. [JL]

In addition, over time, the services themselves became repetitive and unhelp-ful. Laura describes how she would 'sit ... for 1 hour to be seen for 10 minutes, by a different doctor then the last one, and the one before that ... [and] wonder ... why they couldn't review [her] file before calling [her] in'. Once finally in front. Of a service provider, the questions remain the same: 'rate your mood from 1-10 and promise not to kill yourself'. For Laura, this was the only support she felt services provided her.

25.5.3.2. 'Recovery Friends'

As support from services was not enough, participants like Claire and Laura sought out support in the community through peer support groups like the 12-step programme. At these meetings, participant 'g[ot] ... supports ... [and] made new friends' with others 'who had struggled with the same' problems they had. For Laura particularly, 'Even a brief encounter can stay with [her as she felt] understood' [LH].

25.5.4. 'Something to Do, Somewhere to Be, Someone to Talk To'

Due to these supports, the individual finds themselves now on a road to recovery. However, as documented in both the mental health and addiction narratives, recovery is a non-linear process, with an essential element of it being relapse. However, once in active recovery, there are a number of factors that keep them on this road, including being viewed as a person, support from friends and family, volunteering exercise and discharge from services. Fig. 25.14 visually depicts this final phase of a person's recovery journey.

25.5.4.1. Relapse

Despite discovering these arrays of supports, traumatic events can still occur in life, leading to relapse as Claire explains:

> And then I got high. Three years of hard work and I got high ... I was going through some pretty heavy bullying. I started to blame myself. There's something wrong with me. I am the reason I am bullied. How am I hear again. [CF]

However, this time round, participants like Amy could see that this was not her fault, that it was 'just an attempt to regulate [her] emotions' [AR].

25.5.4.2. Recovery

In recovery from a dual diagnosis, the person starts to be viewed as a whole person, not just their addiction or their mental health, but both together as part of a wider system that is the person. In Claire's narrative, she demonstrates this by stating:

> Realising my own experience as someone struggling with a dual diagnosis finally gave me the understanding, I needed to figure out that I could get well. That I could be both an addict and mentally ill and that for me, and maybe others, there was a simple answer in treating both concurrently. With a dual diagnosis its my experience you can't get 'well' without working on both, together.

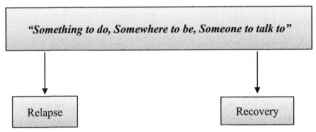

Fig. 25.14.   'Something to Do, Somewhere to Be, Someone to Talk To'.

I wasn't an addict who needed to get clean. I wasn't a lunatic who would never function. I was a whole person who happened to be both and if I addressed both in equal measure I could be ok. [CF]

Another aspect of recovery is support from a person's 'ainm chairde' [AR] or named friends. For Laura, her named friends made a consorted 'effort to reconnect with [her] shortly after [she] moved home'. This made her realise that she 'can't do it alone' [AR], which concluded with Laura realising that she 'wanted to be alive'. In Amy's case, they supported her by 'watching for signs that my mental health is slipping' [AR]. In Laura's case, such supports were beside her as she struggled to maintain her sanity. By using food as a metaphor, her mum described how Laura can get back on track 'one bite at a time'" [LH]. Such a journey to sanity and sobriety is 'a winding road of mistakes and mourning the life I have left behind' [AR]. However, the simplest of things can offer solace to participants as they regain themselves in recovery. For Amy, she 'volunteer[ed her] time [to] helping others who have similar struggles'. For Kate, she swam 'in the sea as often as possible [and did] Yoga once a week'. Laura describes the benefits exercise alone had on her ongoing wellness:

> Running taught me so much about how I understand perseverance, motivation, confidence, when I listen to my head and when to ignore it. Ironically, it gave me a sense of stillness inside myself that I had spent my life seeking through anyone and anything around me. [LH]

Ultimately life in recovery gives individuals the freedom to live 'free from guilt, free from pain' [KB], where one can 'accept ... love knowing [they are] worthy of it' [KB]. All the whilst knowing that they are 'human, [they] have flaws, but [they] don't stop working on improving [them]sel[ves]' [KB].

This realisation also gives individuals the courage to 'make some big changes to [their] routine'. For Laura, this included 'discharge[ing her]self from mental health services' and additionally, as part of her recovery she 'stop[ped] pathologizing every feeling, every thought, and every emotional response' [LH]. For Laura, this 'was a victory [that] just felt right'.

25.6. Conclusion

In summary, from the process of reflexive thematic analysis, three different but interconnecting journeys of recovery were constructed from the 18 narratives in this text. Each journey began with a traumatic event and a series of compounding factors that made these traumatic events more likely to have a negative impact on the person's development over time. This led to a period of suffering, trying to fit in, but ultimately leads to further isolation and feelings of shame and guilt that leads to self-harm and suicidal ideation resulting in the involvement of services. Once services become involved, they offer a diagnosis, followed by pharmacological interventions with no other support. This leads individuals to gradually discover their own supports within their communities and as a result enter a phase of active recovery, which sometimes can lead to relapse. However, the person is more prepared this time for the return of these negative emotions and cravings and as such, utilises their support to regain recovery and a life of their own choosing.

References

Braun, V., & Clarke, V. (2006). Using thematic analysis in psychology. *Qualitative Research in Psychology, 3*(2), 77–101.

Braun, V., & Clarke, V. (2019). Reflecting on reflexive thematic analysis. *Qualitative Research in Sport, Exercise and Health, 11*(4), 589–597. https://doi.org/10.1080/21 59676X.2019.1628806

Braun, V., & Clarke, V. (2022). *Thematic analysis: A practical guide.* SAGE Publications Ltd.

Jacob, K. S. (2015). Recovery model of mental illness: A complementary approach to psychiatric care. *Indian Journal of Psychological Medicine, 37*(2), 117–119. https://doi.org/10.4103/0253-7176.155605

Norton, M. J. (2021). Co-production in child and adolescent mental health: A systematic review. *International Journal of Environmental Research and Public Health, 18*(22), 11897. https://doi.org/10.3390/ijerph182211897

Norton M. J., & Flynn, C. (2021). The evidence base for wellness recovery action planning (WRAP): A protocol for a systematic literature review and meta-analysis. *International Journal of Environmental Research and Public Health, 18*(24), 13365. https://doi.org/10.3390/ijerph182413365

Chapter 26

Recommendations as it Relates to Policy, Practice and Service Users

Oliver John Cullen[a] and Michael John Norton[b]

[a]*HSE Mental Health Services, Ireland*
[b]*HSE Office of Mental Health Engagement and Recovery, Ireland*

Abstract

From the process of reflexive thematic analysis in the previous chapter, three models of recovery were constructed. Each model had a number of similarities in terms of phases, but also had several differentials that made each journey in their own way unique. This chapter builds on the work of the previous chapter by providing a number of recommendations aimed towards policy, service providers and service users in an attempt to improve the service that those with a mental health, addiction or dual diagnosis challenge may require and experience in the future.

Keywords: Recommendations; policy; service users; stakeholders; practice

26.1. Introduction

In the previous chapter, through the process of reflexive thematic analysis, three interconnecting journeys of recovery were constructed. Each had a number of similarities to one another along with several differential factors. As a result of the process of reflexive thematic analysis, it has become clear that the construction of these journeys has implications across services and those stakeholders that are involved in them. As such, this chapter aims to lay out a set of recommendations that can support those reading, as well as policymakers to understand

Different Diagnoses, Similar Experiences:
Narratives of Mental Health, Addiction Recovery and Dual Diagnosis, 207–210
Copyright © 2024 by Oliver John Cullen and Michael John Norton
Published under exclusive licence by Emerald Publishing Limited
doi:10.1108/978-1-80455-848-520241026

the interconnectivity of mental health, addiction and dual diagnosis. To do this, Section 26.2 will discuss recommendations as they relate to policy in this area. This is followed by recommendations relating to the work of both mental health and addiction professionals in Section 26.3. Following which, Section 26.4 lays out recommendations for the service user with a mental health, addiction or dual diagnosis challenge as it relates to their unique recovery journey. Section 26.5 concludes this chapter with a synopsis of what has been discussed. What follows is a discussion on the recommendations as they relate to policy.

26.2. Recommendations for Policy

Policy has the power to change practices as the need arises within society. With the ever-increasing evidence base regarding mental health, addiction and dual diagnosis, policy change and its subsequent implementation can play an important part role in implementing research meaningfully into practice for the benefit of all in service provision. The following recommendations in this text come from real-world examples from 18 brave voices who have experienced a mental health, addiction or dual diagnosis challenge and have volunteered to tell us their unique story. The recommendations that follow will give credence to those narratives.

Recommendation 1: Ensure appropriate mechanisms are put in place in order to treat co-occurring disorders, that these mechanisms are given the priority and sensitivity required to assist individuals in receiving the best possible outcome from the service they draw support from.

Recommendation 2: Ensure proper, evidence-based training structures are put in place as per the best available international evidence, to support service providers and their organisations to carry out their daily tasks in an informed, educated and timely manner. This, in turn, would take pressure from service provision as the right support and treatment option are applied based on good practice and the best available evidence.

From the findings of this text, it is clear that a number of additional training mechanisms are needed for inclusion in the mandatory training list that service providers are duty and legally bound to complete as per their employment. Such training should include:

- Trauma informed practice.
- Addiction training for mental health service providers. To support the rollout of training based on the best available evidence, policymakers must ensure that funding is allocated to service as required.

Recommendation 3: Continue to invest, develop and support initiatives based on lived experience, peer support, recovery education and local forums, as these mechanisms are essential for the recovery process at a micro, meso and macro level to occur.

26.3. Recommendations for Mental Health and Addiction Professionals

This book recognises the practice of wisdom, knowledge, expertise and passion from service providers. This book has identified the recovery processes of individuals with mental health, addiction and dual diagnosis challenges, and the role of service providers along that journey of recovery. The following recommendations are provided to support service providers in journeying through recovery with the service providers based on the eighteen narratives in this text.

Recommendation 1: As a 'service provider' ask yourself, is this a service I want for my loved ones. Have I listened to that person? Have I understood and valued their experiences? Can I approach that individual or family member in a trauma informed and empathetic manner, all the while respecting their core values and beliefs? From the narratives reviewed in this text, it seems that this was not always the case. As such, service providers could engage in Recovery Principles as part of their training regimens so that the importance of this is emphasised and embedded in their practices.

Recommendation 2: Service providers should become aware of and become sensitive to the phenomena of dual diagnosis. From this text, we have gathered that, such challenges are transfigurations of a traumatic experience and its associated pain. In the case of dual diagnosis, asking for help can prove challenging. Service providers should support these individuals in a manner that serves to support their additional needs and not re-traumatise them.

Recommendation 3: The key to success in many interactions can be education and listening. When the right education practices are in place, it gives a structure that allows the service provider to learn. As mentioned within the recommendations for policy, additional training is required in a number of areas including trauma informed practice. To support such training, services should, when clinically safe to do so, provide individual service providers with protected time and funding to support reflection and additional educational needs that can be of benefit to the entire service, including for service users and not just the individual service provider in question.

26.4. Recommendation for Service Users

For the individual who may read this book and enquire how this will impact their own recovery, a series of recommendations are now presented to support you in understanding what may be applicable to your own life. Recovery is a non-linear, ever-evolving process. As such, these recommendations may guide or complement your own personal recovery journey. These recommendations are as follows.

Recommendation 1: As outlined above, recovery is a non-linear journey with many peaks and troughs. Relapse is usually part of that process. Despite this, relapse can also serve a distinct purpose in re-evaluation. Particularly as it relates to what went wrong? What triggered it? And what changes you can make in order to grow, learn from mistakes and develop new paths to support your recovery. Relapse can be used as an educative tool to re-align your values and perspectives and in turn, make you more aware and prepared for future challenges. As such, you as a service user should use relapse, not as a wipe to punish oneself for not maintaining recovery, but rather use it as a stepping stone to learn from past mistakes and grow in your recovery.

Recommendation 2: Your diagnosis, trauma and circumstances do not define you. You are defined by your resilience, awareness and the positive people within your life that love, encourage and support you no matter what. 'Stick with the winners' and reach out to others who may be struggling to find their recovery path and offer support when you can.

Recommendation 3: As individuals seeking to embrace recovery, personal responsibility should be on the top of your list. The journey of recovery is about finding oneself in an ever-evolving landscape and that comes with autonomy and personal responsibility. 'You alone can do it, but you can't do it alone'. Embrace recovery. The contributors to this book have embraced recovery and have found solace within that journey that cannot be found elsewhere. Finally, an important part of recovery is finding your voice, which can provide you with an opportunity to be a part of service change. Co-production within services (see Chapter 5), through initiatives like the local forums, help to reduce stigma through conversation that can also serve as a key to change within service provision.

26.5. Conclusion

In summary, we have provided a list of recommendations based on the 18 narratives for policy, service providers and service users. Although this is not an exhaustive list, it serves as a starting point for scholars, policymakers and other interested parties to begin discussions on this important issue. The chapter that follows will conclude this text while keeping in mind the above recommendations in order to support and encourage stakeholders to develop these issues further, so that those struggling can get the best possible support they require regardless of class, economic status or geographical location.

Part 6

Concluding Remarks

Chapter 27

Conclusions and Sign Posting

Oliver John Cullen[a] and Michael John Norton[b]

[a]*HSE Mental Health Services, Ireland*
[b]*HSE Office of Mental Health Engagement and Recovery, Ireland*

Abstract

This, the final chapter of the text, provides the reader with a synopsis of the chapters that have gone before and concludes with a list of helpful resources for the reader, most of which is based in an Irish context. Although this remains a contentious issue in service provision, it is hoped that this book and the narratives within demonstrate the close relationship between mental health, addiction and dual diagnosis.

Keywords: Recovery; society; co-production; service user involvement; policy

27.1. Introduction

This concluding chapter gives a brief synopsis of the material discussed in previous chapters. It provides a list of helpful resources and offers encouragement for individuals in recovery to continue on this path. This encouragement comes from the 18 contributors' narratives, which demonstrate courage and resilience that is made possible for all as they sought a life in recovery. The listed supports provided at the end of the chapter is to be used as a source of education and support for all stakeholders, inclusive of service users, family members/friends and supporters. For practitioners, these resources should provide them with options of support to individuals and/or supporters they interact with.

Different Diagnoses, Similar Experiences:
Narratives of Mental Health, Addiction Recovery and Dual Diagnosis, 213–215
Copyright © 2024 by Oliver John Cullen and Michael John Norton
Published under exclusive licence by Emerald Publishing Limited
doi:10.1108/978-1-80455-848-520241027

27.2. Brief Summary and Reflections

The following is a brief summary of each of the chapters of this text.

- *Chapter 1*, 'Contextual and Personal Introduction to the Text' explored the conceptual and cultural exploration of mental health, addiction and dual diagnosis.
- *Chapter 2*, 'Mental Health, Addiction and Dual Diagnosis: National and International Policy' reflected on three healthcare systems of various jurisdictions and their bespoke policies for mental health, addiction and dual diagnosis.
- *Chapter 3*, 'Recovery in Mental Health, Addiction and Dual Diagnosis' introduced 'recovery' as a concept within the traditional services and explored some of the baseline models that are used within.
- *Chapter 4*, 'The Conundrum of Dual Diagnosis' presented the multifaceted and complex issue of co-occurring disorders, in the context of mental health and addiction.
- *Chapter 5*, 'Co-production and the Lived Experience Perspective' described the inclusion of lived experience as an integral part of the process of reform in the challenges outlined within the context of the book. It delineated the value of co-production as a process of empowering lived experience as a core foundation of knowledge.
- *Chapter 6*, 'The Challenges of Mental Health, Addiction and Dual Diagnosis in an Irish Context' puts forward the cultural impact of mental health, addiction and dual diagnosis in an Irish context, and explores how in recent decades there has been a shift in mindset in terms of the approach to the treatment of mental health addiction and dual diagnosis.
- *Chapters 7–24* discuss contributors narratives of mental health, addiction and dual diagnosis.
- *Chapter 25*, 'Fusing Experiences, Reflexive Thematic Analysis' describes the results of the process of reflexive thematic analysis. It identified similarities and differences between the recovery journeys of mental health, addiction and dual diagnosis.
- *Chapter 26*, 'Recommendations as it Relates to Policy, Practice and Service Users' expands on the previous chapter by providing a list of recommendations as it relates to three important areas of service provision. These areas are policy, practice and the end user. Such recommendations serve not as an exhaustive list but as a catalyst for conversations to begin/continue in this area of service provision.

27.3. Helpful Resources

1. Recovery College, Dublin North/North East; https://recoverycollege.ie
2. Recovery College South East; https://www.recoverycollegesoutheast.com
3. Recovery College West; https://www.recoverycollegewest.ie
4. Arches Recovery College; https://archesrecovery.ie
5. Shine; https://shine.ie

6. Grow Mental Health; https://shine.ie
7. Mental Health Engagement and Recovery; https://www.hse.ie/eng/services/list/4/mental-health-services/mental-health-engagement-and-recovery/
8. Pieta; https://www.pieta.ie/how-we-can-help/helpline/
9. Samaritans; https://www.samaritans.org/ireland/samaritans-ireland/
10. Better Together; https://serdatf.ie/bettertogether/
11. Family Addiction Support Network; https://fasn.ie
12. Family Support Network; https://www.peerfamilysupport.org
13. Drug information/support; http://www.drugs.ie
14. Teac Tom; https://www.thethomashayestrust.com
15. Dual Diagnosis Ireland; https://www.dualdiagnosis.ie
16. St Patrick's University Hospital; https://www.stpatricks.ie
17. St John of God Hospital; https://stjohnofgodhospital.ie
18. Smarmore Castle; https://www.smarmore-rehab-clinic.com
19. Narcotics Anonymous Ireland; https://www.na-ireland.org
20. Alcoholics Anonymous Ireland; https://www.alcoholicsanonymous.ie
21. Lifering; https://lifering.ie
22. Smart Recovery; https://smartrecovery.ie
23. Rape Crisis support; https://www.rapecrisishelp.ie
24. Involvement Centre; https://www.involvementcentres.com
25. Mental Health Ireland; https://www.mentalhealthireland.ie

Printed and bound by CPI Group (UK) Ltd, Croydon, CR0 4YY

14/08/2024

14540999-0001